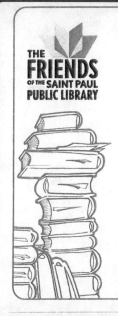

FLOWERS

A Collection of Floral Photography
and Proverbial Wisdom

An Interactive Book for Memory-Impaired Adults

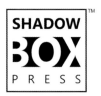

Shadowbox Press books are designed to facilitate a rewarding reading experience by providing entertainment, education, and comfort to individuals diagnosed with Alzheimer's disease, Parkinson's disease, stroke, brain injury, or other memory-impairment condition.

For more information, go to www.shadowboxpress.com

Shadowbox Press, established in 2009, is an independent publisher committed to providing high-quality, interactive books to the memory-impaired adult audience.

Published by Shadowbox Press, LLC
P.O. Box 268
Richfield, OH 44286
www.shadowboxpress.com

Chief Creative Director: Matthew Schneider
Product Development Director: Deborah Drapac, BSN, RN

This book is intended to be informational and should not be considered a substitute for advice from a health care professional. The authors and the publisher expressly disclaim responsibility for any adverse effects arising from the use or application of the information contained in this book.

Publisher's Cataloging-in-Publication data

Schneider, Matthew John.
    Flowers : a collection of floral photography and proverbial wisdom, an interactive book for memory-impaired adults / Matthew Schneider ; Deborah Drapac, BSN, RN.
    p. cm.
    ISBN-13: 978-0-9831577-4-8; ISBN-10: 0-9831577-4-X
1. Alzheimer's disease—Patients—Rehabilitation. 2. Dementia—Patients—Rehabilitation.
3. Caregivers. 4. Self-care, Health. I. Drapac, Deborah Ann. I. Title.

RC523.S37 2011
362.196'831—dc22   2010917061

Manufactured in China

FLOWERS

A Collection of Floral Photography
and Proverbial Wisdom

An Interactive Book for Memory-Impaired Adults

Matthew Schneider
Deborah Drapac, BSN, RN

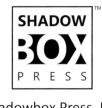

Shadowbox Press, LLC
Richfield, Ohio

INTRODUCTION

Shadowbox Press began with one simple mission: to develop interactive products for memory-impaired adults to revisit and share memories through the reading experience.

Storytelling is a valuable form of communication that connects one another and allows us to relate to each other on a personal level. It sparks the imagination, promotes self-reflection, and provides a way to find meaning in our experiences.

We have published a collection of books that offer a variety of subject matter designed to engage the user with meaningful content and provide a connection to both the past and present. Every effort has been made in the development of these books to maximize the experience for the user. They may be read independently or shared with an individual by a caregiver, loved one, staff member, or volunteer.

Our books offer a rewarding reading experience that stimulates the mind and offers engagement opportunities for the user. You will find inspiring words, inviting photographs, innovative conversation prompts, and unique activities to facilitate an interactive, multi-sensory experience. These books can generate meaningful communication and provide the feeling of well-being associated with sharing experiences and stories together. Through engagement, you may discover common backgrounds and interests, realize mutual bonds, and/or participate in a quality conversation.

We believe the reading experience should be shared at all stages of life, and sincerely hope that our passion for books touches your heart. We trust that you will find meaning, delight, and comfort in sharing a title from our collection of Shadowbox Press books. May you explore and discover memories, share experiences, and reflect on the value and purpose of life.

At Shadowbox Press, we welcome feedback from our readers and listeners. Please contact us at www.shadowboxpress.com to share your reading experiences, stories, and suggestions for future books.

ABOUT THIS BOOK

This book has been created to provide an interactive reading experience for a memory-impaired adult. It is designed to encourage socialization, evoke memories, prompt conversation, and supply mental and physical stimulation, thereby improving the overall quality of life for the individual user.

There are a variety of benefits from using this book. By encouraging engagement through personal reminiscing; a feeling of empowerment, an elevated mood, a positive self-image, and/or a reduced level of depression may result. In addition, a caregiver's presence, support, and attention can communicate acceptance, reassurance, and affection to a memory-impaired adult.

This book is comprised of three sections:

1. The STORY is the foundation of the book and is designed to entertain, inform, inspire, and/or educate. It features inviting photographs paired with engaging, large-print text written in clear, concise, and easy-to-read sentences. The content is intended to cultivate an interest in reading, evoke memories, and encourage opportunities to reminisce.

2. CONVERSATION STARTERS are questions that directly correlate to an individual set of pages from the STORY. Each series of inquiry-based questions are designed to prompt a dialog from experiences, events, and/or relationships. Engaging in conversation provides a memory-impaired adult the opportunity to share special memories and unique experiences from their life.

3. ACTIVITIES are exercises based on sensory stimulation, creative expression, and physical movement. These simple but purposeful activities correspond to the overall theme of the book, and are designed to provide additional mental and physical enrichment. Participation in a variety of activities is essential to overall good health and emotional well-being.

This book does not have to be read in its entirety to provide a benefit. Each set of pages is intended to encourage thinking, stimulate emotions, and evoke unique memories. An individual page may trigger a response and lead to a meaningful conversation. Through the reading and reminiscing process, the user can share his or her unique life story, express personal values, and, perhaps, reveal a legacy to pass on to future generations.

INTERACTION GUIDELINES

Communication is what connects us to each other. Because memory impairment slowly diminishes communication skills, it creates distinct challenges in how an individual communicates their thoughts and emotions, as well as comprehend what is being communicated to them. The key to managing the behaviors associated with memory impairment lies in the methods of engagement by caregivers and others. It is important to adapt our thinking and behaviors to create a more comfortable environment for a memory-impaired adult.

Guidelines for a successful reading experience:

- Locate a quiet, comfortable setting, free of distractions, for the reading experience.
- Before beginning, take a moment and allow yourself to relax. Imagine a connection between the voice and the story and reflect upon the importance of the time spent together.
- Always approach the individual from the front and make eye contact.
- Position your head at the same level as the individual's head. Bend your knees or sit down to reach a correct level.
- Smile whenever it's appropriate. A connection can grow from a smile.
- Present the book to the individual and invite them to share in the reading experience.
- Read aloud slowly, in an adult tone with a clear, calm, inviting, and enthusiastic voice, pausing after each sentence.
- Speak in short, direct sentences, focusing on a single idea at a time.
- Focus on central words and ideas, emphasizing the ones that may evoke memories.
- Point out key aspects of the photographs and invite the individual to share their thoughts.
- Include your own comments and encourage the individual to share their memories by prompting them with the CONVERSATION STARTERS.
- Ask only one question at a time, allowing the individual to answer it before continuing.
- Be aware of nonverbal cues. It is often possible to recognize a connection by observing facial expressions and/or body language.
- After a response, either verbal or nonverbal, acknowledge the contribution with positive reinforcement and encourage further discussion.
- Remember to be patient, as it may take longer for a memory-impaired adult to fully process and respond to a particular word, phrase, idea, or image.
- At times, engagement may become challenging. However, always treat the individual with dignity and respect.

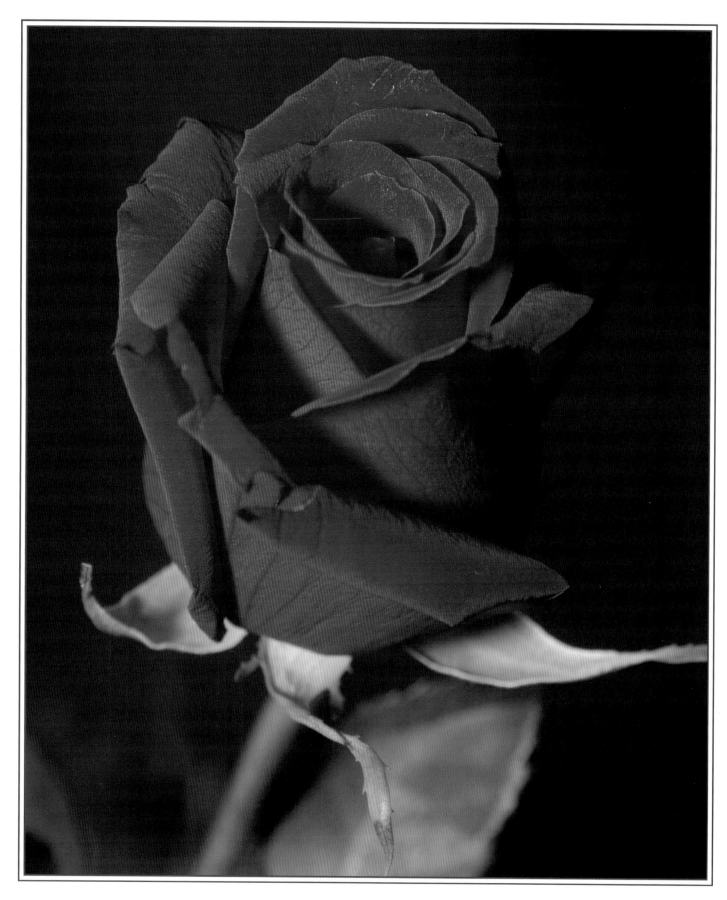

Rose

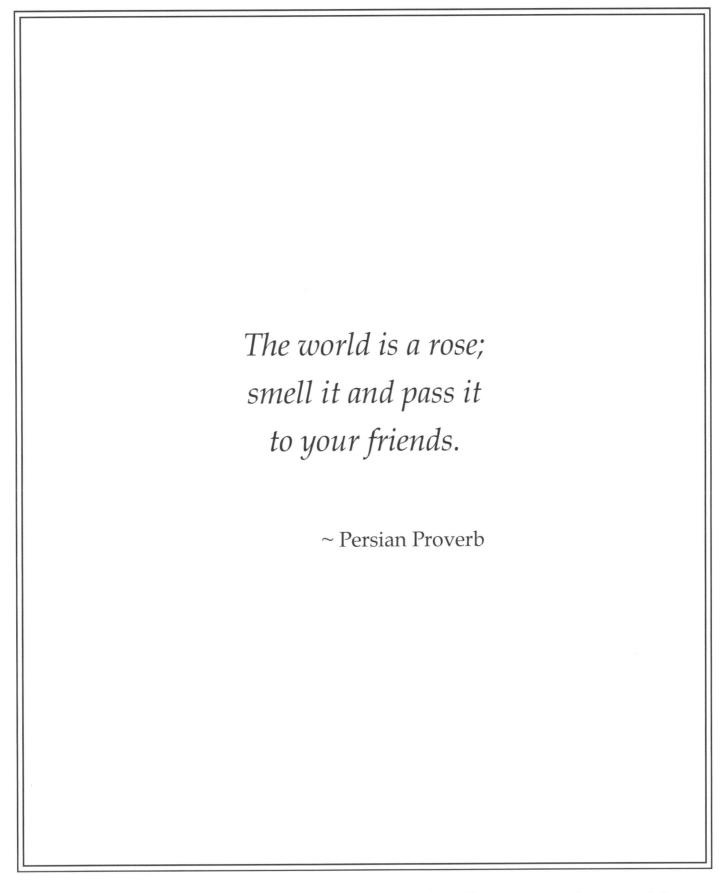

The world is a rose;
smell it and pass it
to your friends.

~ Persian Proverb

Roses are considered the most popular flowers in the world.

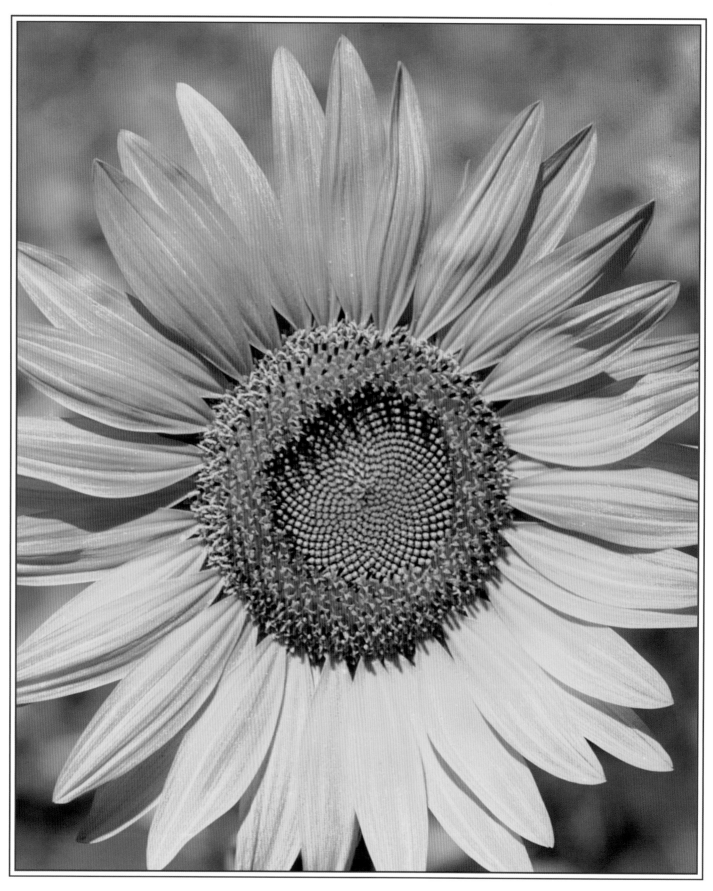

Sunflower

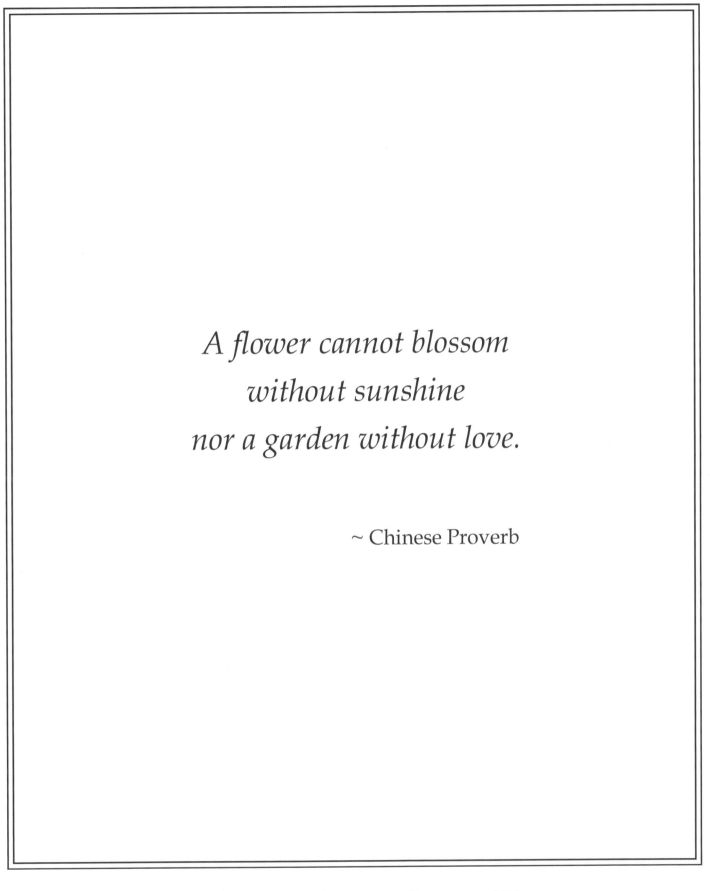

A flower cannot blossom
without sunshine
nor a garden without love.

~ Chinese Proverb

The sunflower is the state flower of Kansas.

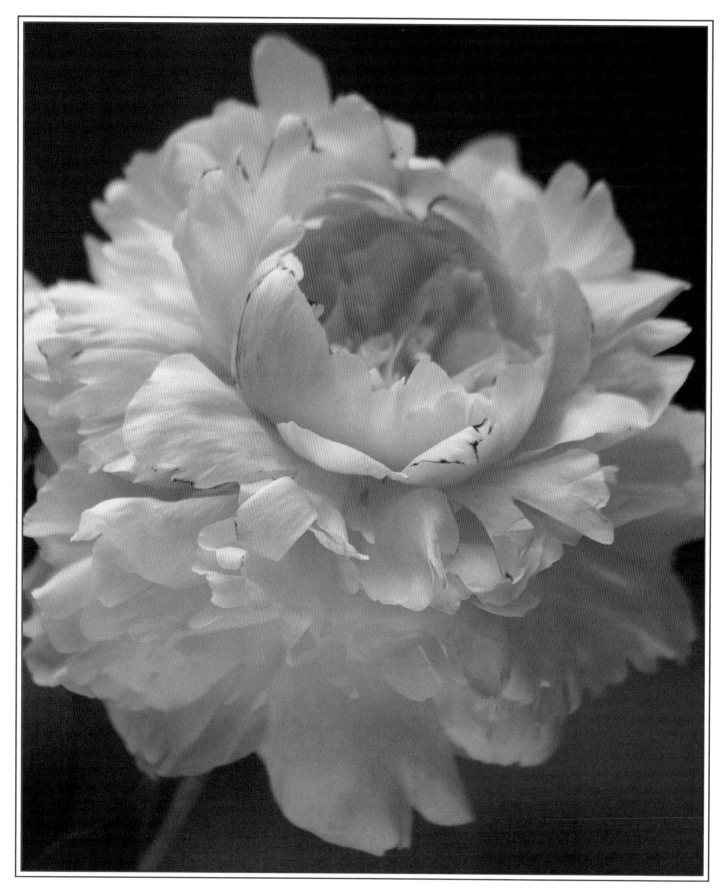

Peony

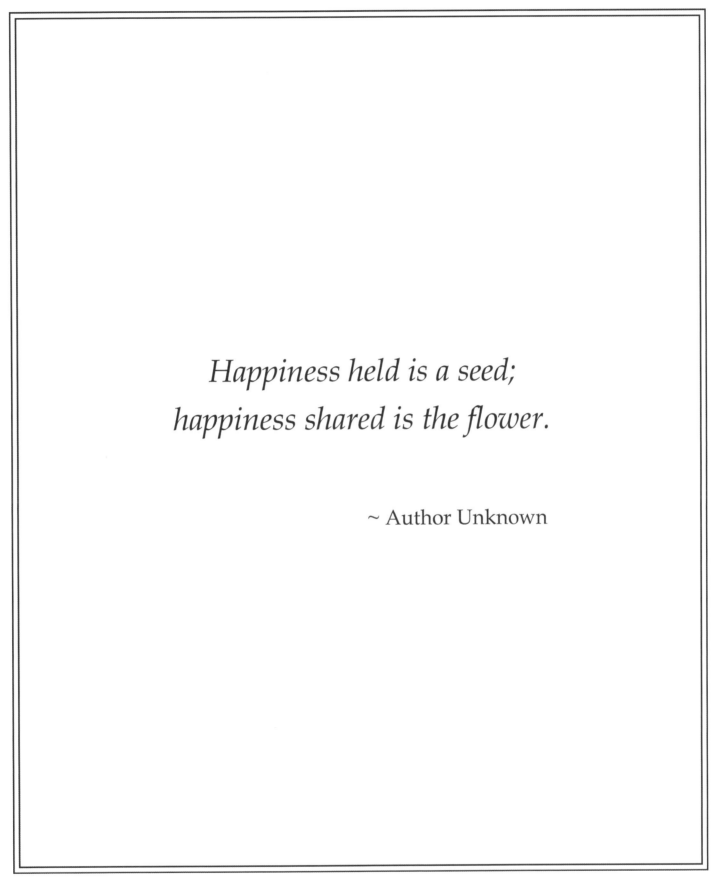

Happiness held is a seed;
happiness shared is the flower.

~ Author Unknown

Peonies are regarded as symbols of wealth, luck, and happiness.

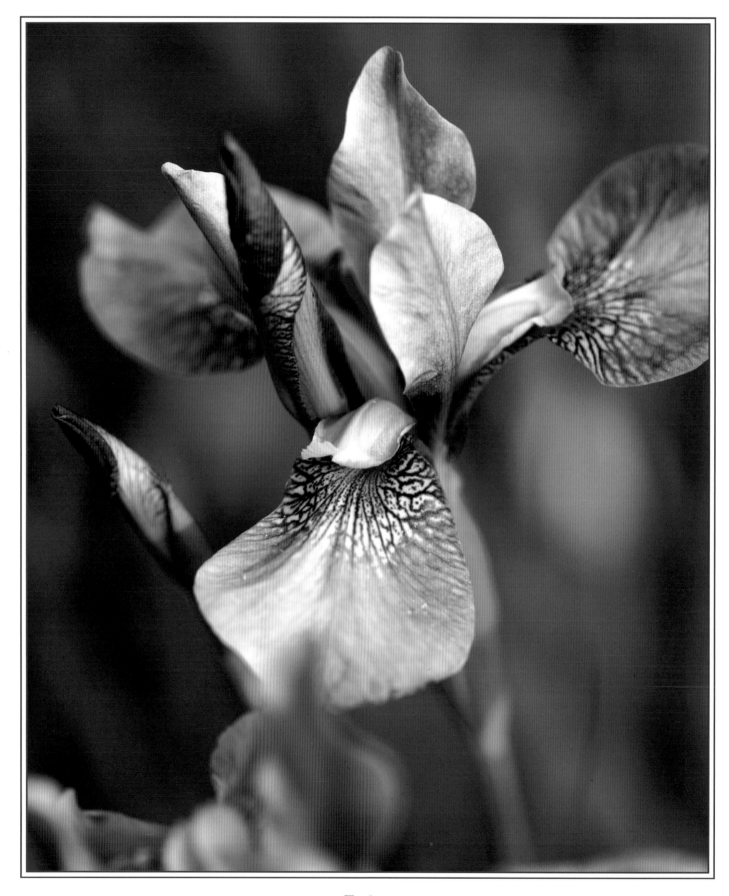

Iris

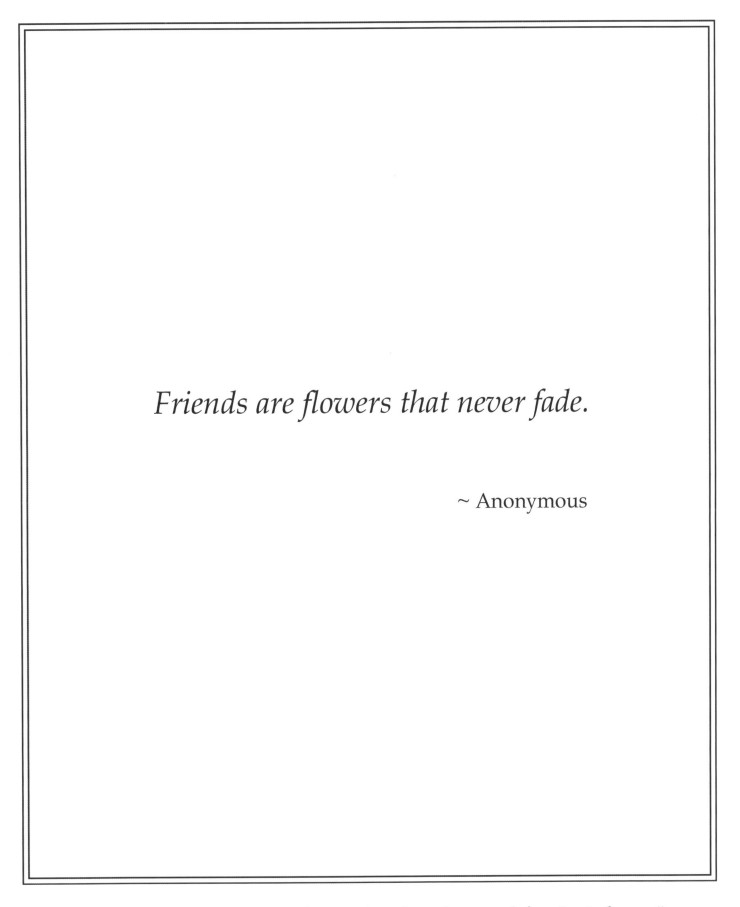

Friends are flowers that never fade.

~ Anonymous

The iris gets its name from the Greek word for "rainbow."

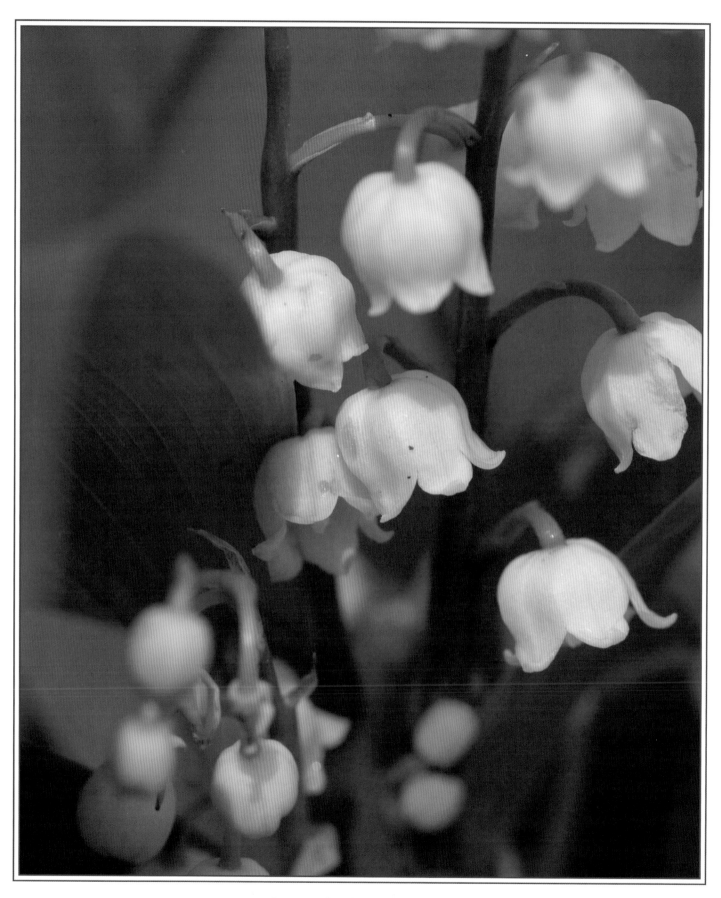

Lily of the Valley

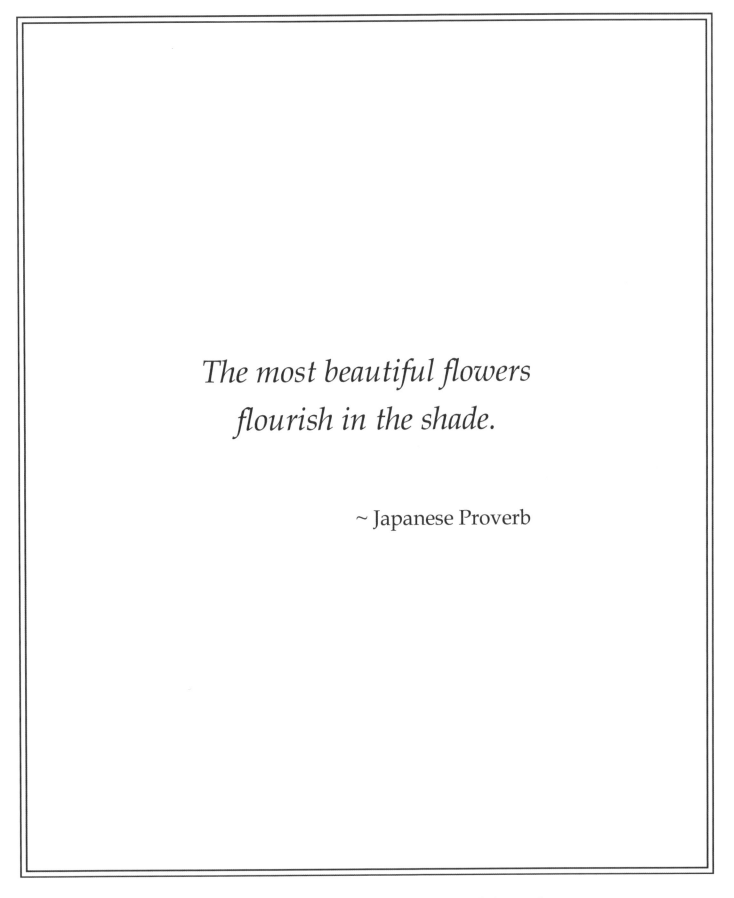

The most beautiful flowers
flourish in the shade.

~ Japanese Proverb

Lily of the valley is often used in wedding bouquets.

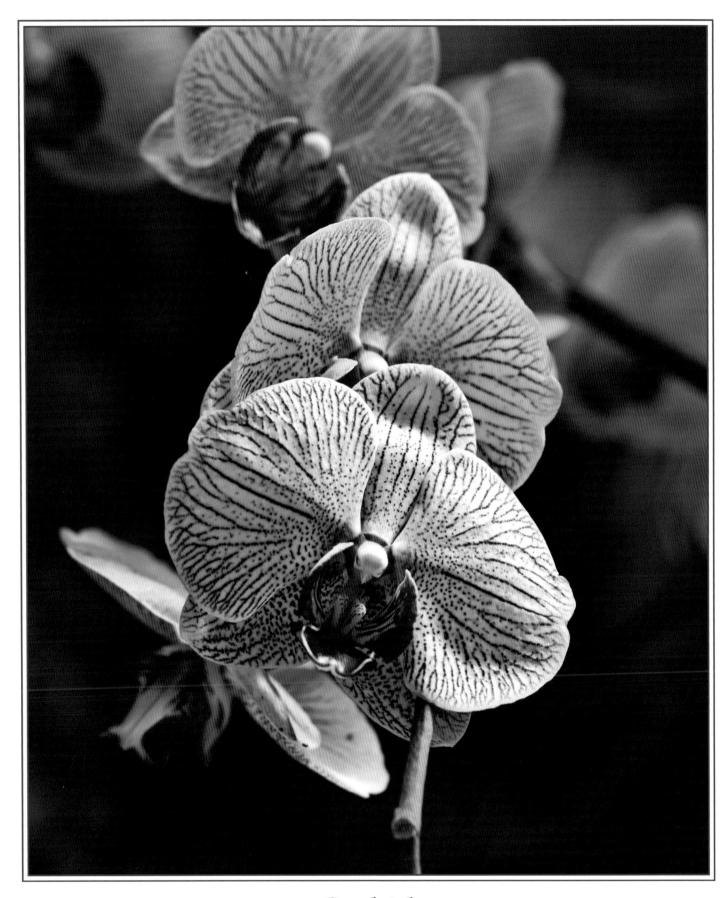

Orchid

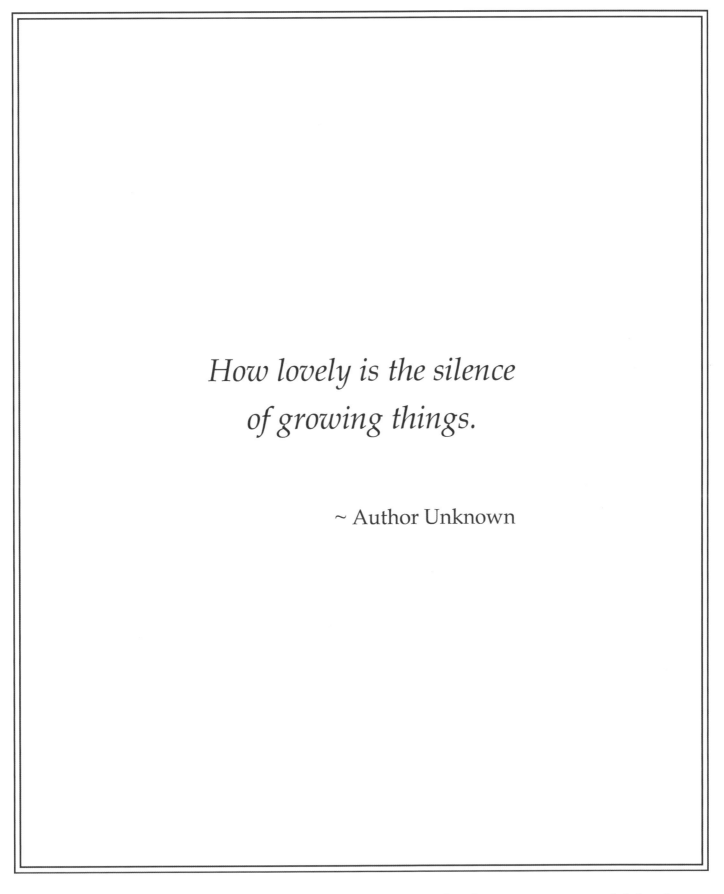

How lovely is the silence
of growing things.

~ Author Unknown

Orchids come in a variety of colors, including green and black.

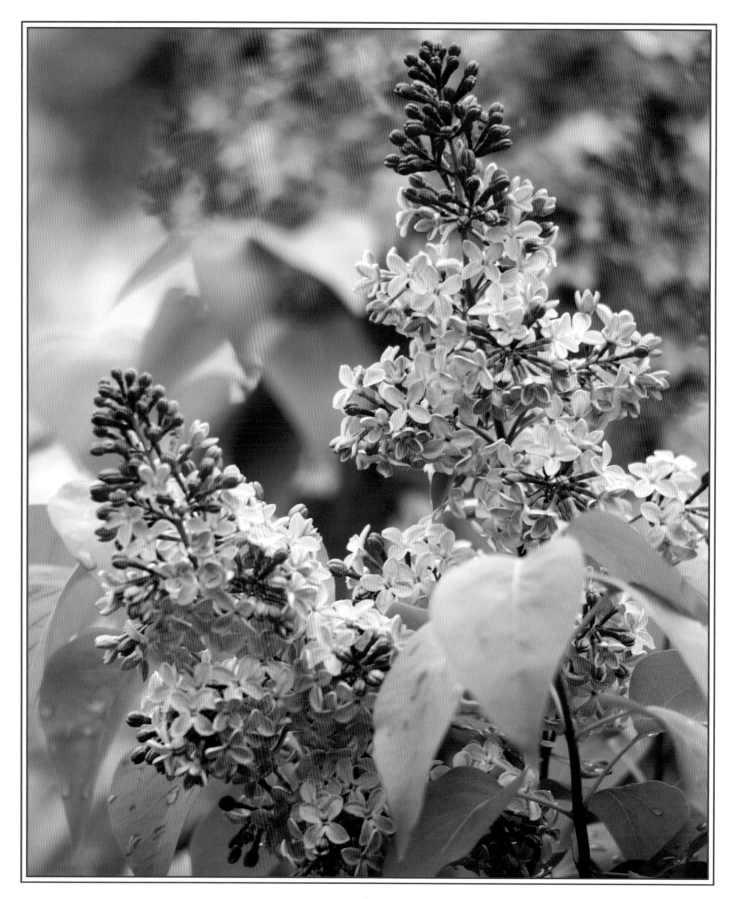

Lilac

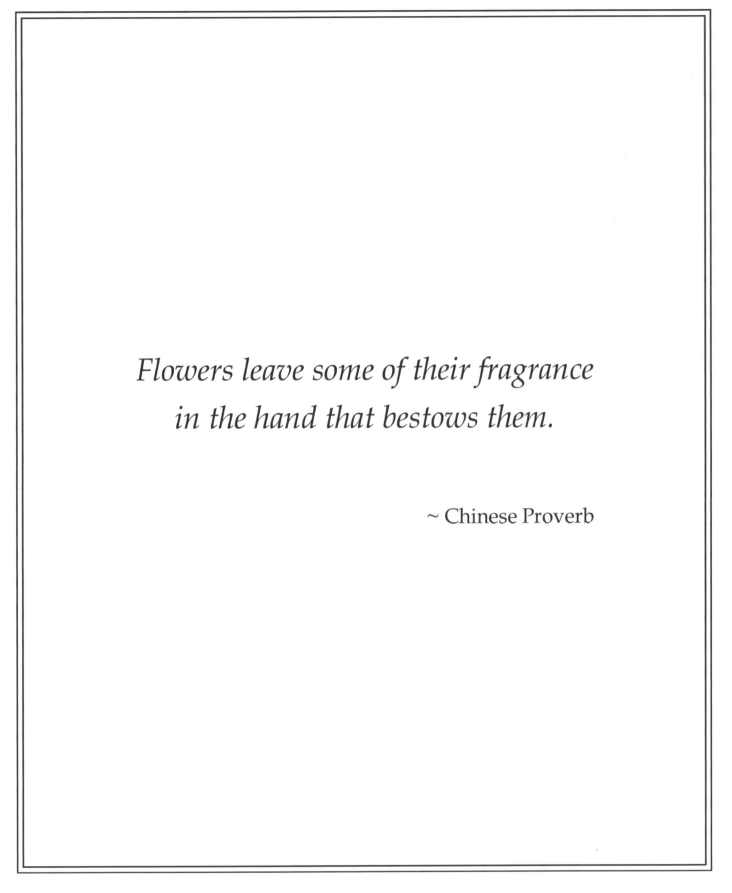

*Flowers leave some of their fragrance
in the hand that bestows them.*

~ Chinese Proverb

Lilac bushes can live for hundreds of years.

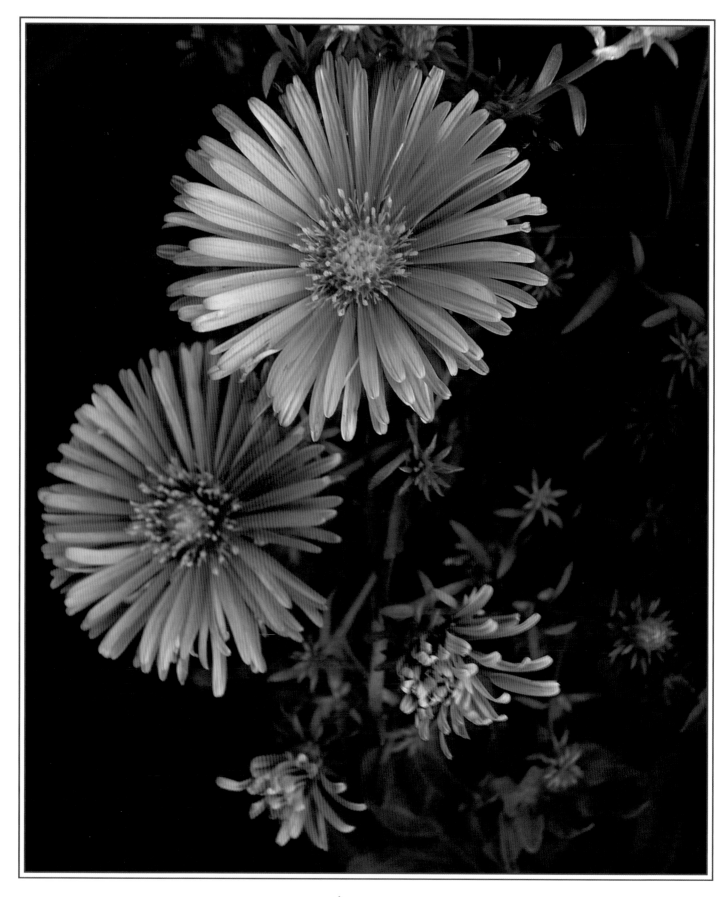

Aster

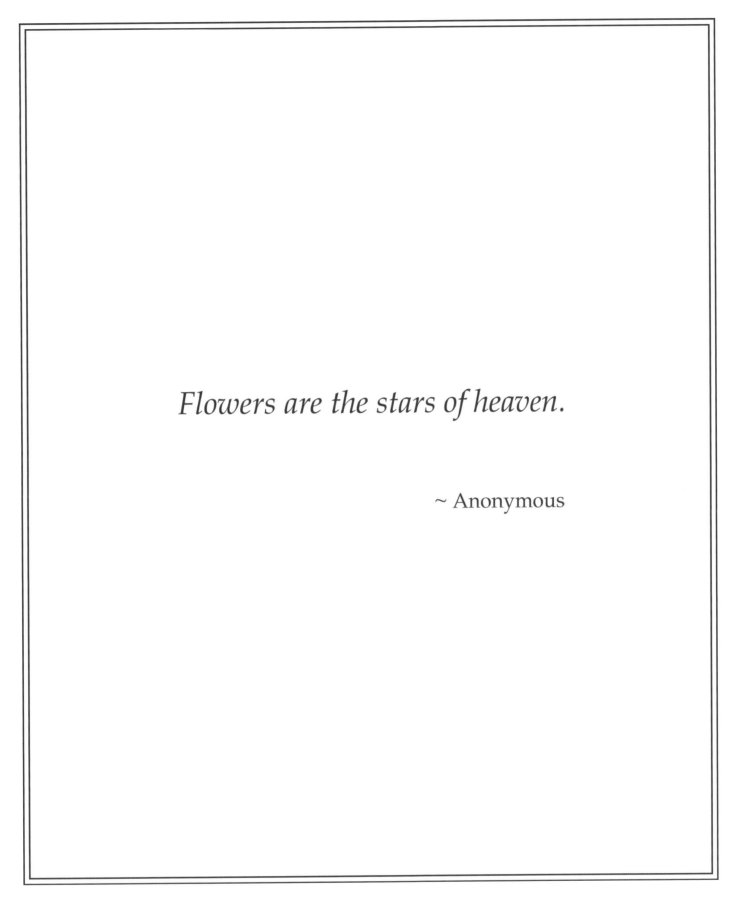

Flowers are the stars of heaven.

~ Anonymous

Asters generally bloom in late summer and early fall.

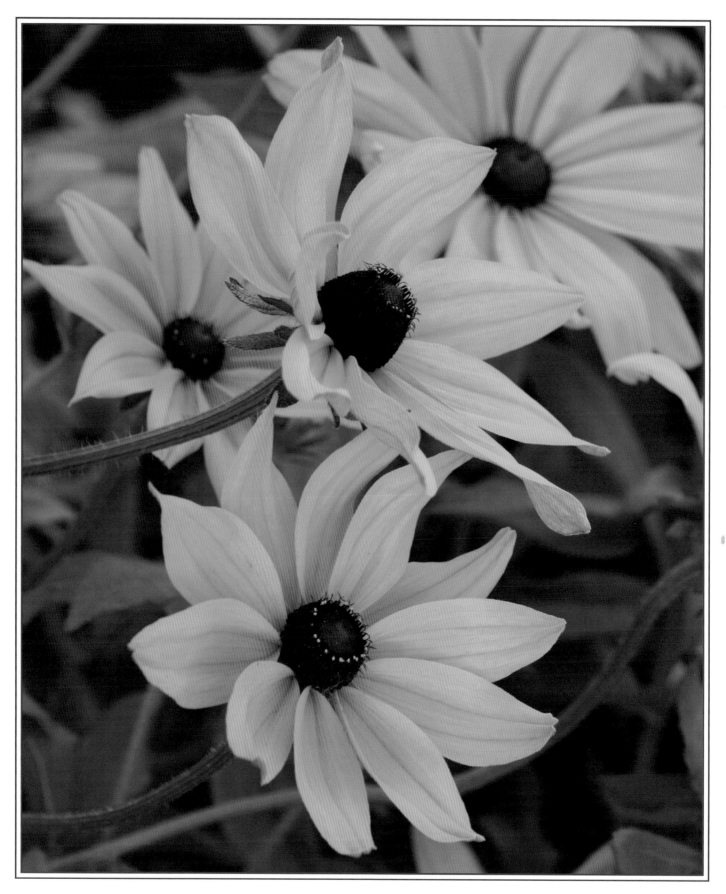

Black-Eyed Susan

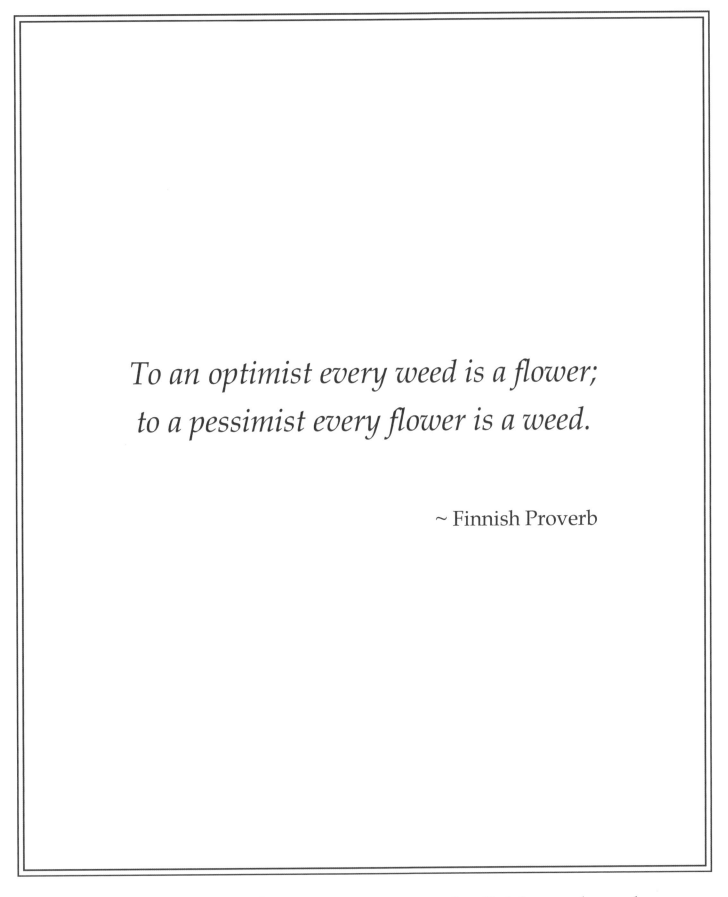

To an optimist every weed is a flower;
to a pessimist every flower is a weed.

~ Finnish Proverb

Black-eyed Susans thrive in open woods, fields, and gardens.

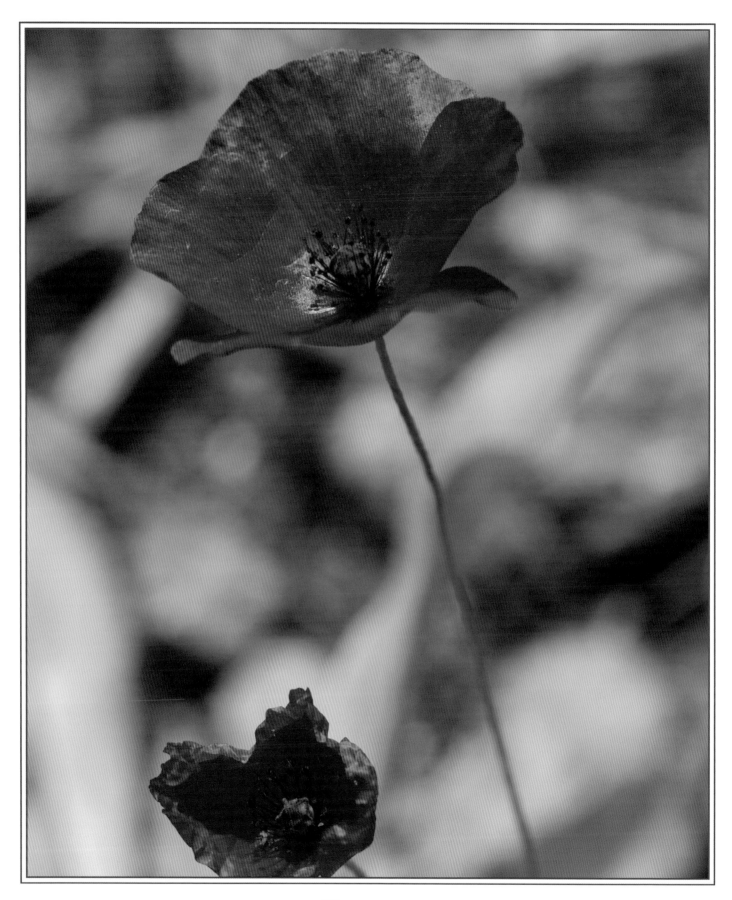

Poppy

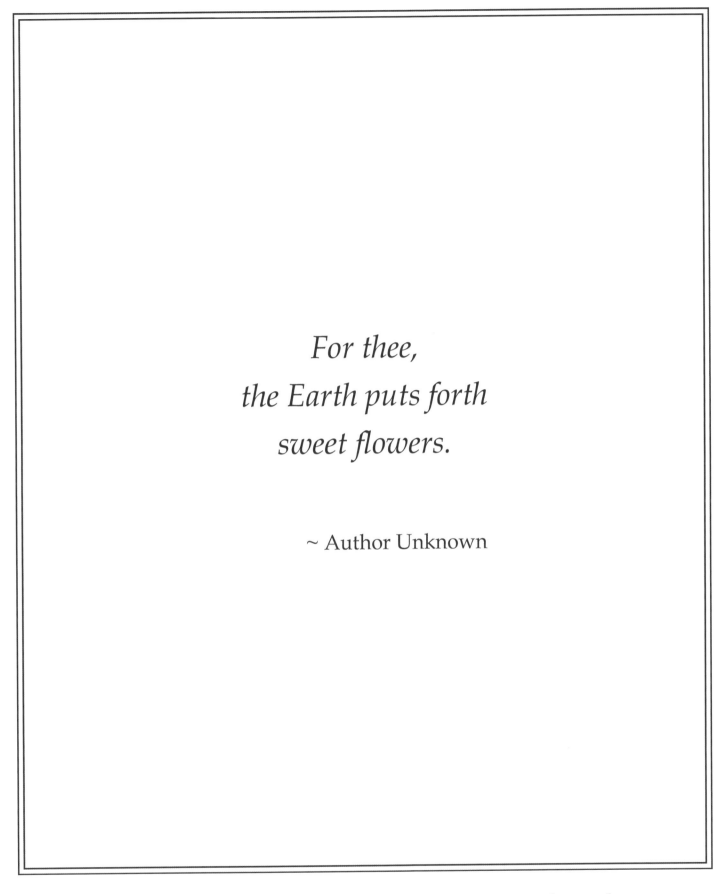

For thee,
the Earth puts forth
sweet flowers.

~ Author Unknown

Poppies have delicate, crepe paper-textured petals.

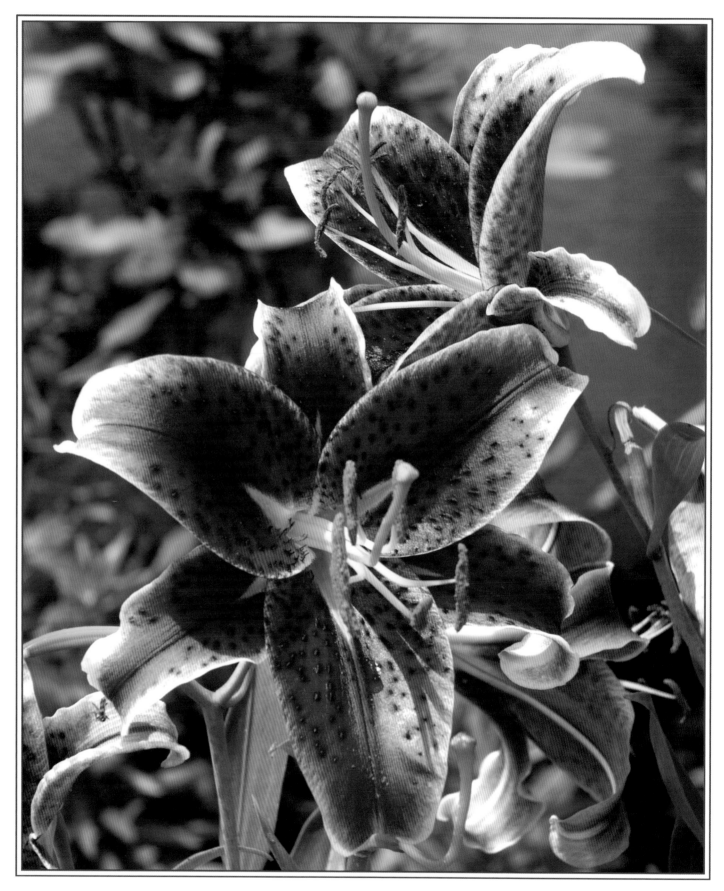

Lily

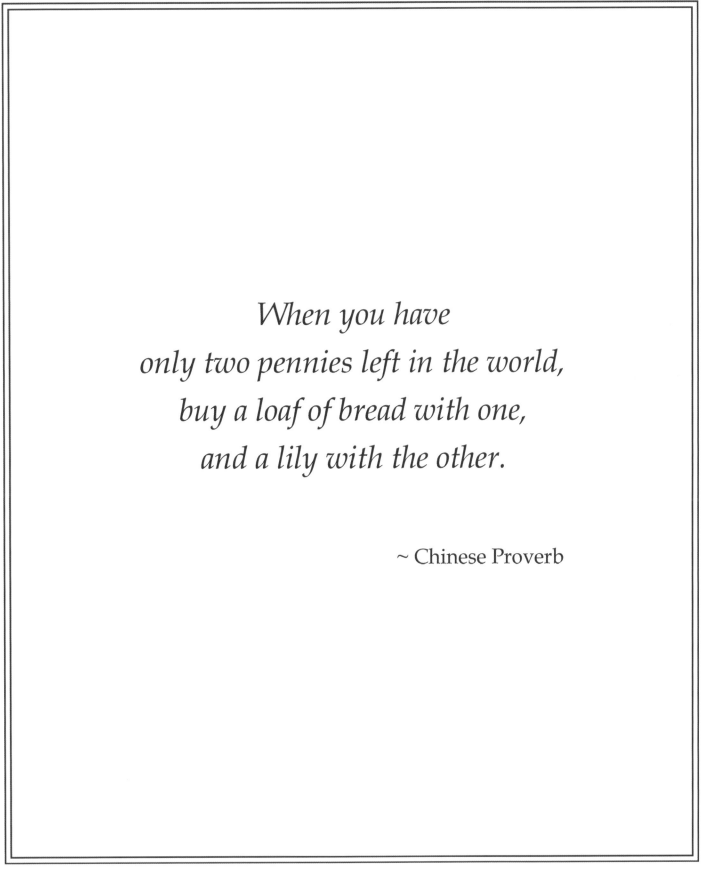

When you have
only two pennies left in the world,
buy a loaf of bread with one,
and a lily with the other.

~ Chinese Proverb

Lilies have been cultivated for over 3,000 years.

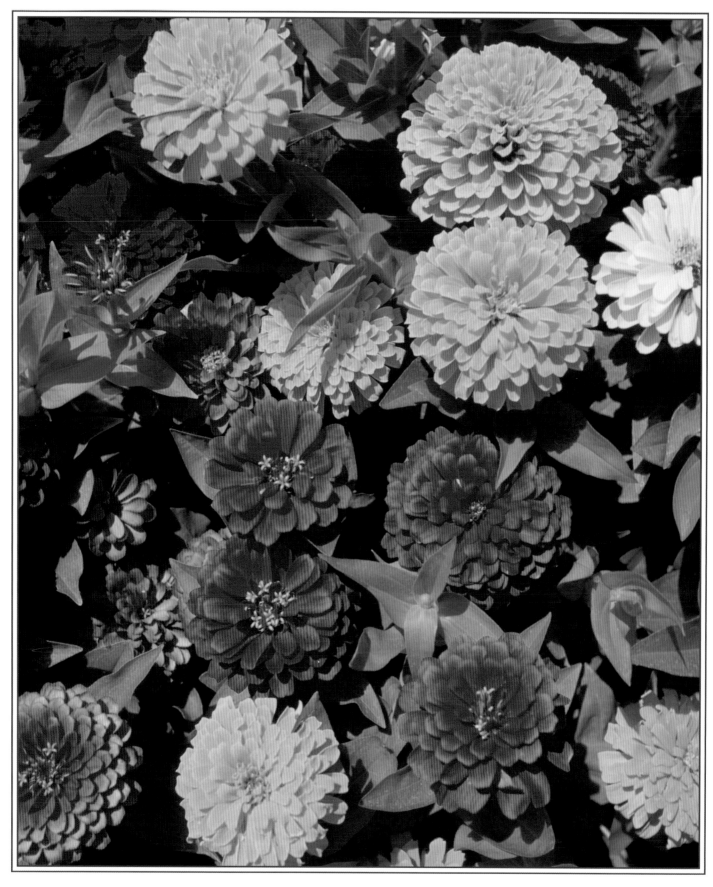

Zinnia

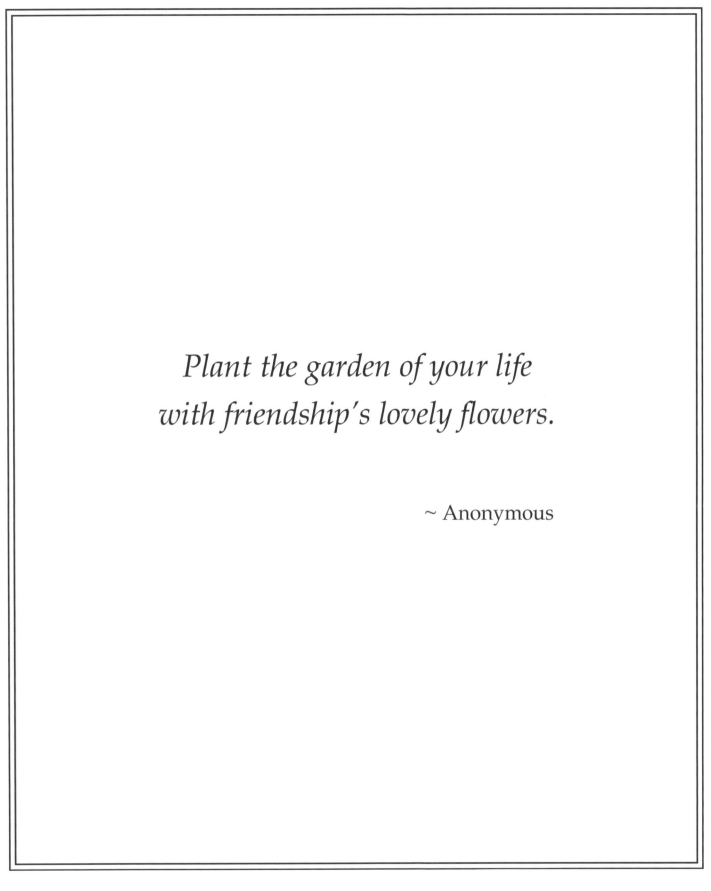

*Plant the garden of your life
with friendship's lovely flowers.*

~ Anonymous

Zinnias are vibrant flowers that love high heat and strong sunlight.

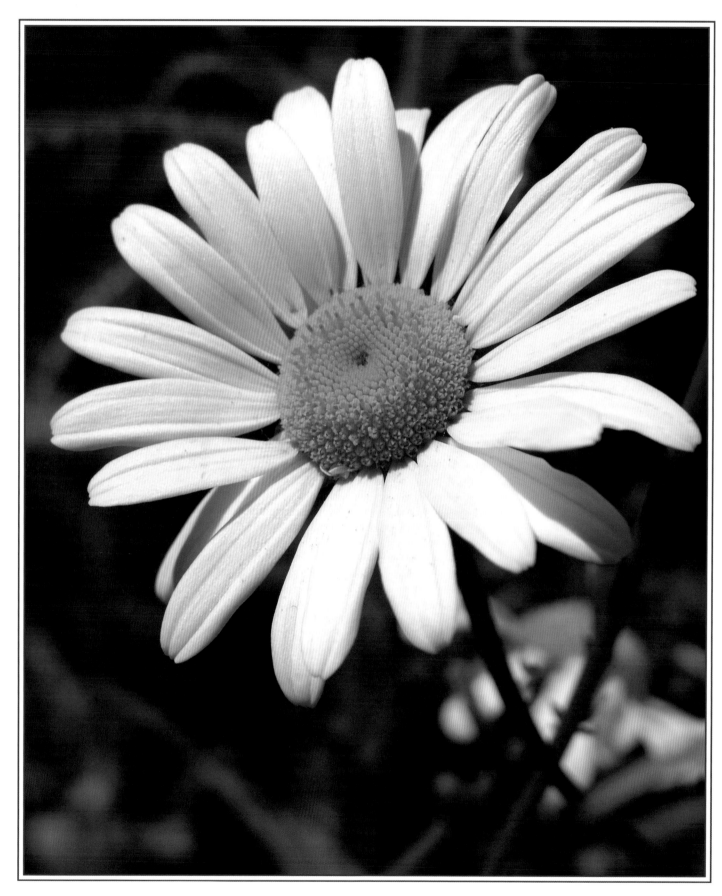

Daisy

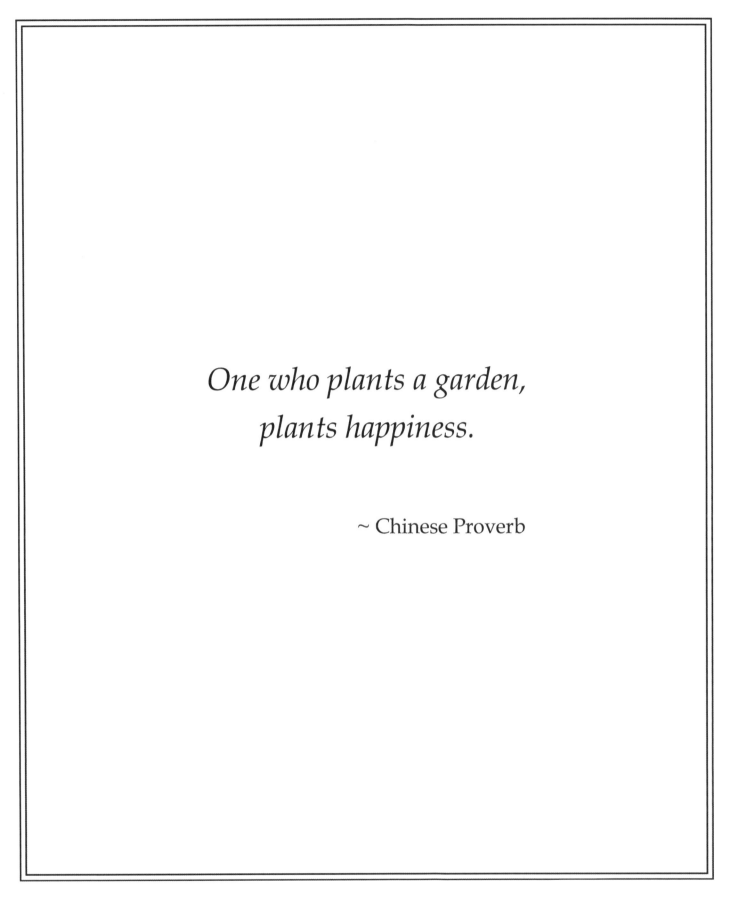

One who plants a garden,
plants happiness.

~ Chinese Proverb

The daisy is the birthday flower for April.

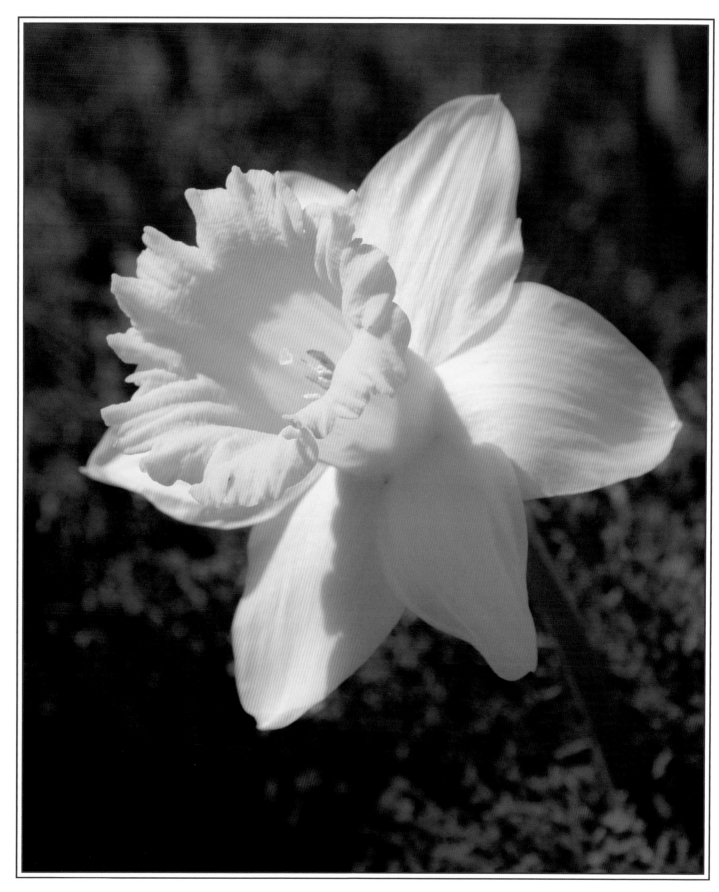

Daffodil

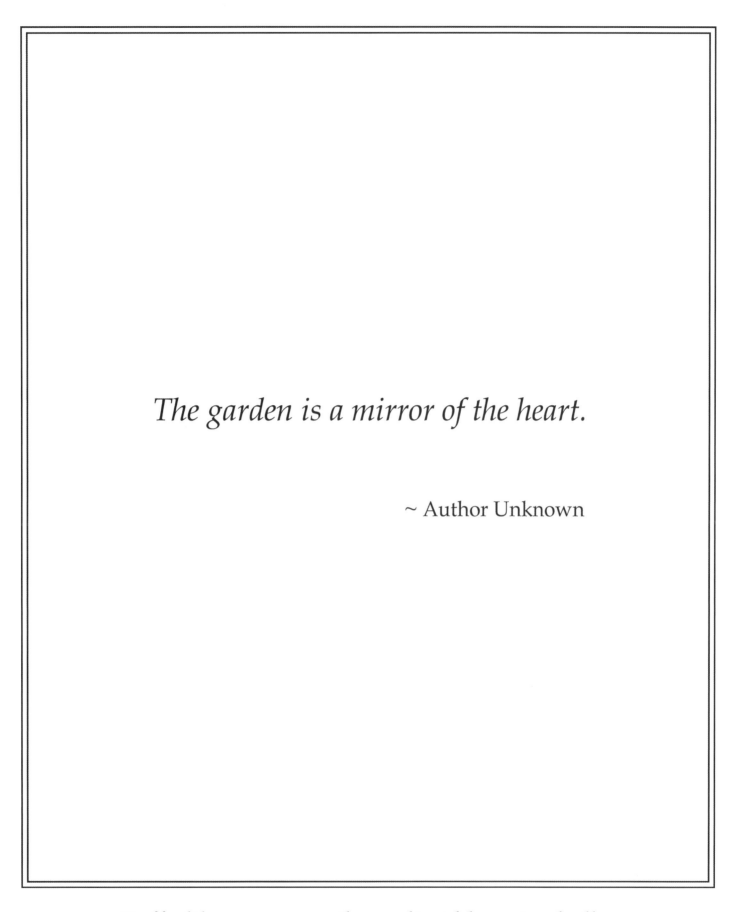

The garden is a mirror of the heart.

~ Author Unknown

Daffodils are among the earliest blooming bulbs.

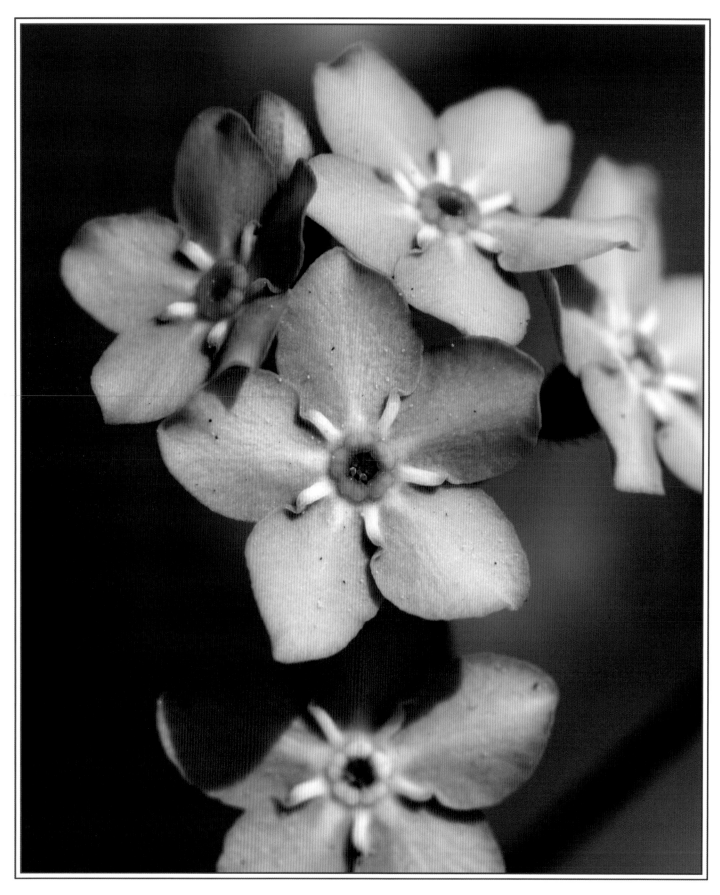

Forget-Me-Not

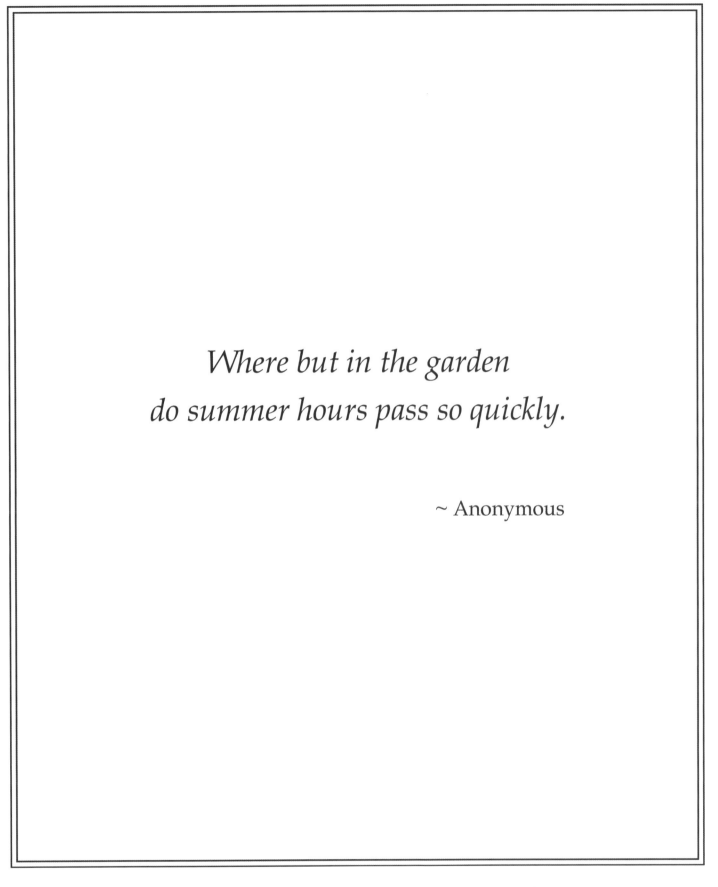

Where but in the garden
do summer hours pass so quickly.

~ Anonymous

Forget-me-nots are native to Europe and Asia.

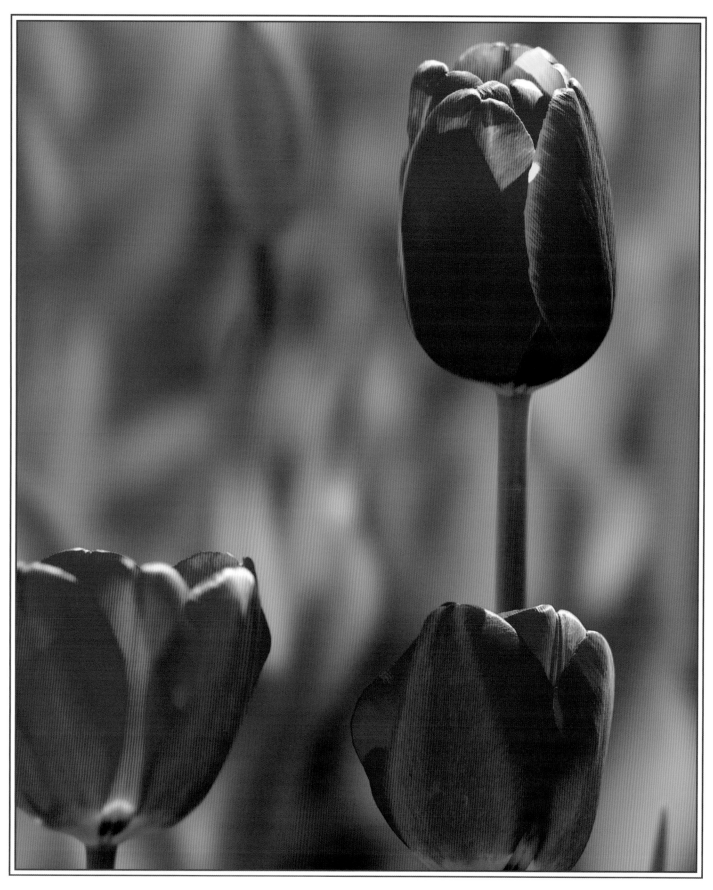

Tulip

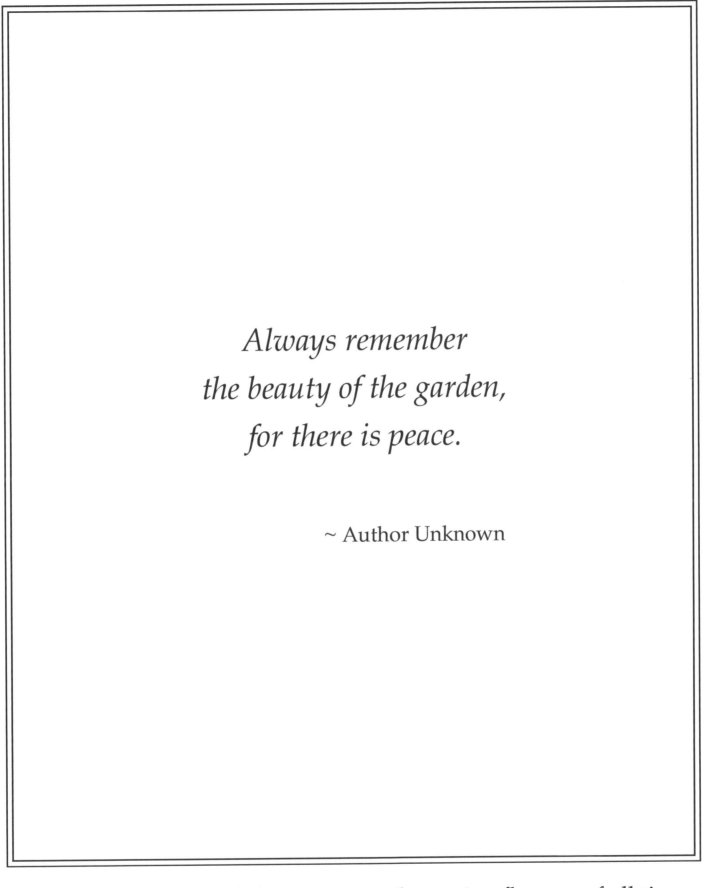

*Always remember
the beauty of the garden,
for there is peace.*

~ Author Unknown

Tulips are considered the most popular spring flowers of all time.

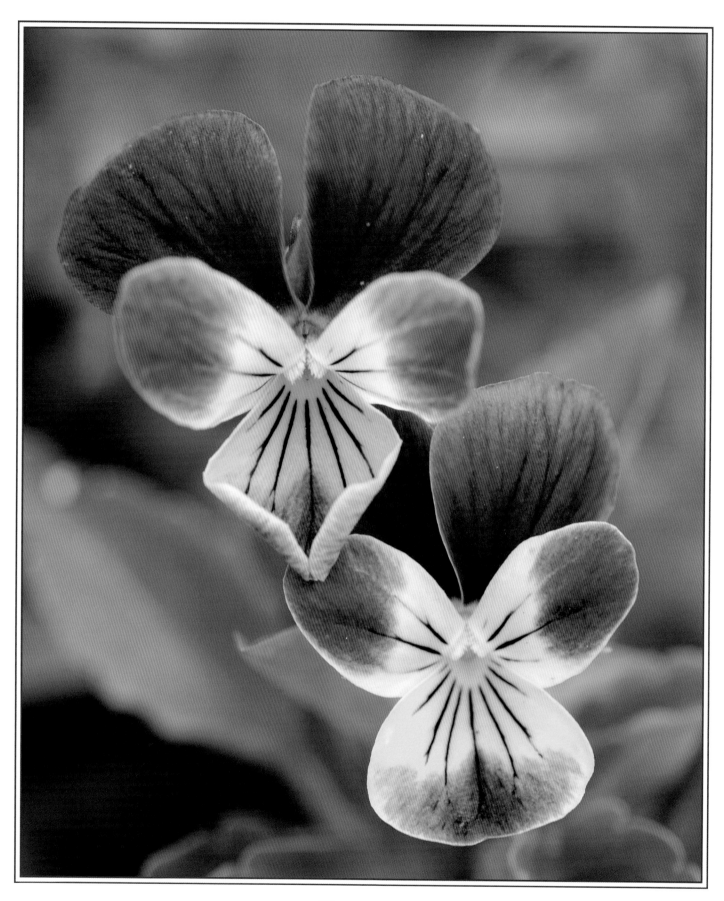

Pansy

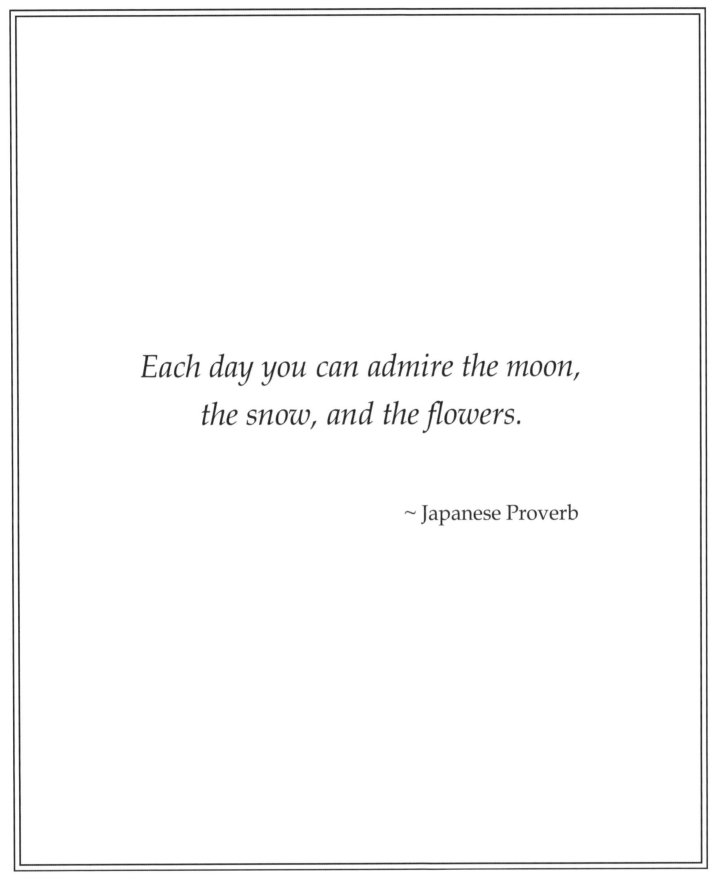

Each day you can admire the moon,
the snow, and the flowers.

~ Japanese Proverb

Pansies have a delicate perfume-like aroma.

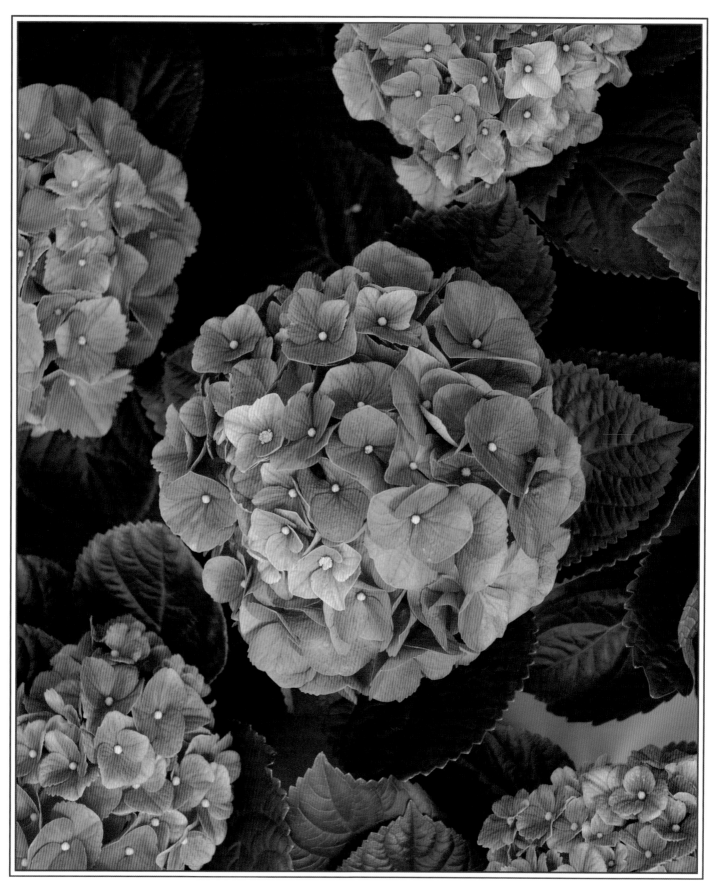

Hydrangea

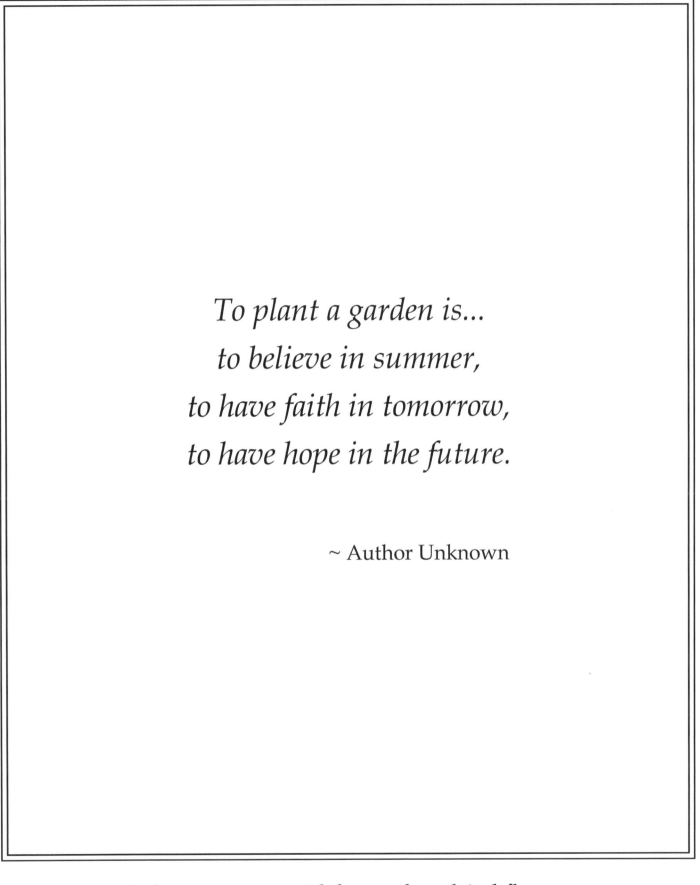

To plant a garden is...
to believe in summer,
to have faith in tomorrow,
to have hope in the future.

~ Author Unknown

Hydrangeas are widely used as dried flowers.

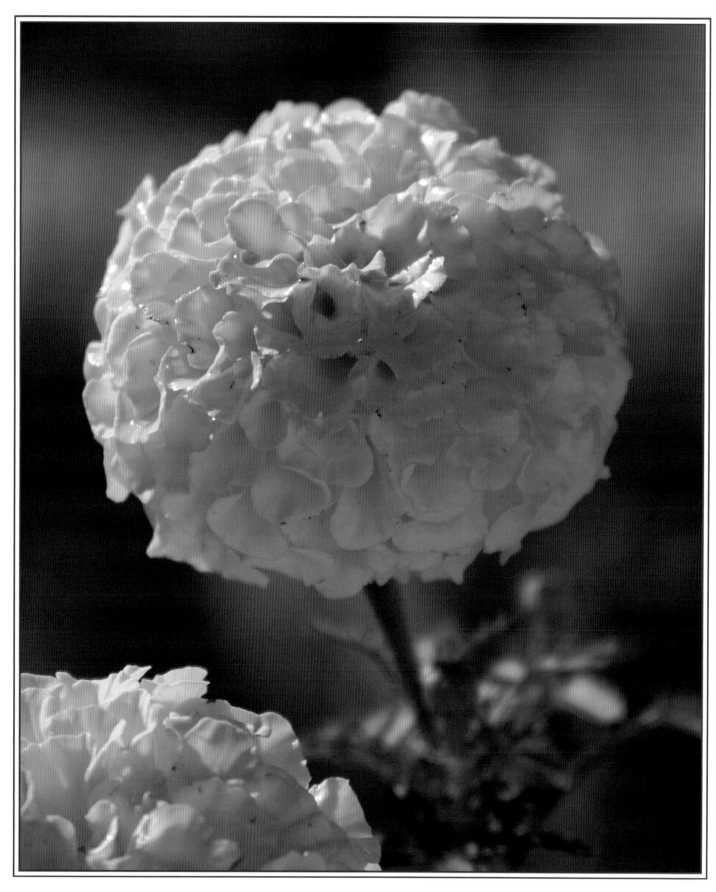

Marigold

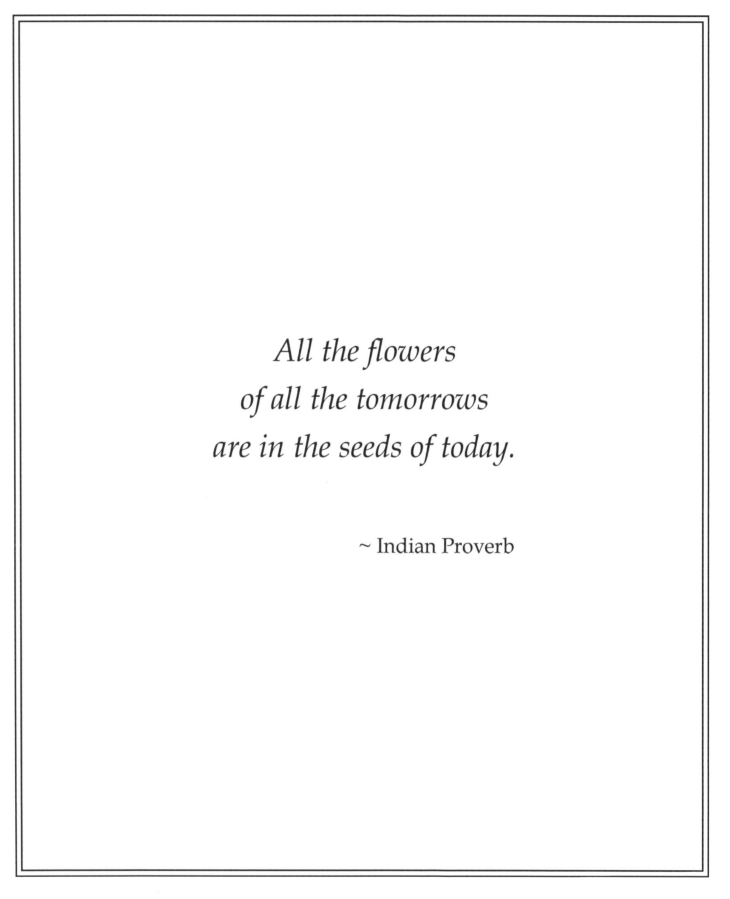

All the flowers
of all the tomorrows
are in the seeds of today.

~ Indian Proverb

The musky, pungent scent of marigolds repels harmful insects.

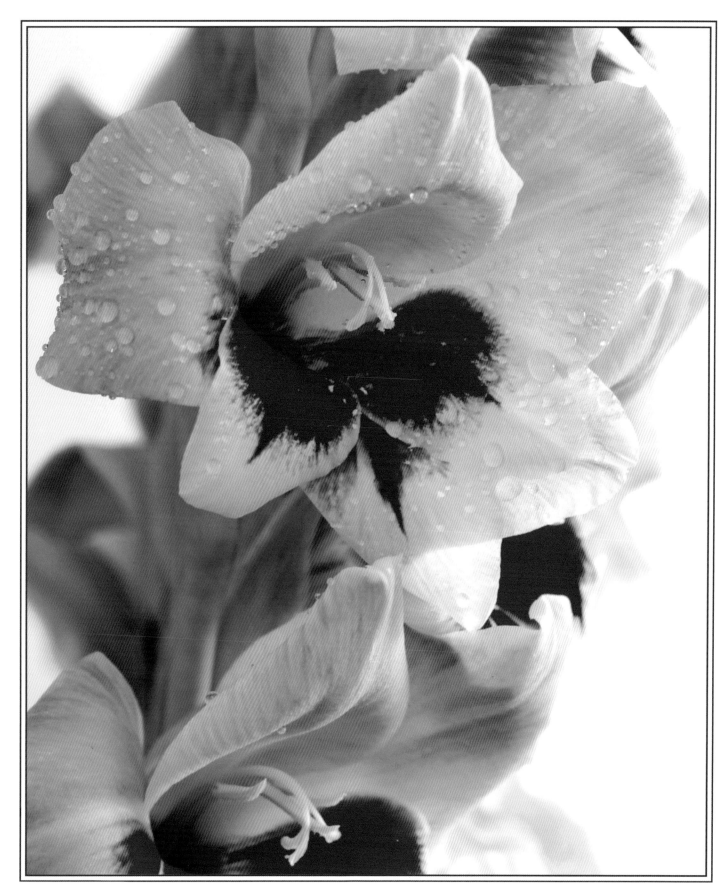

Gladiolus

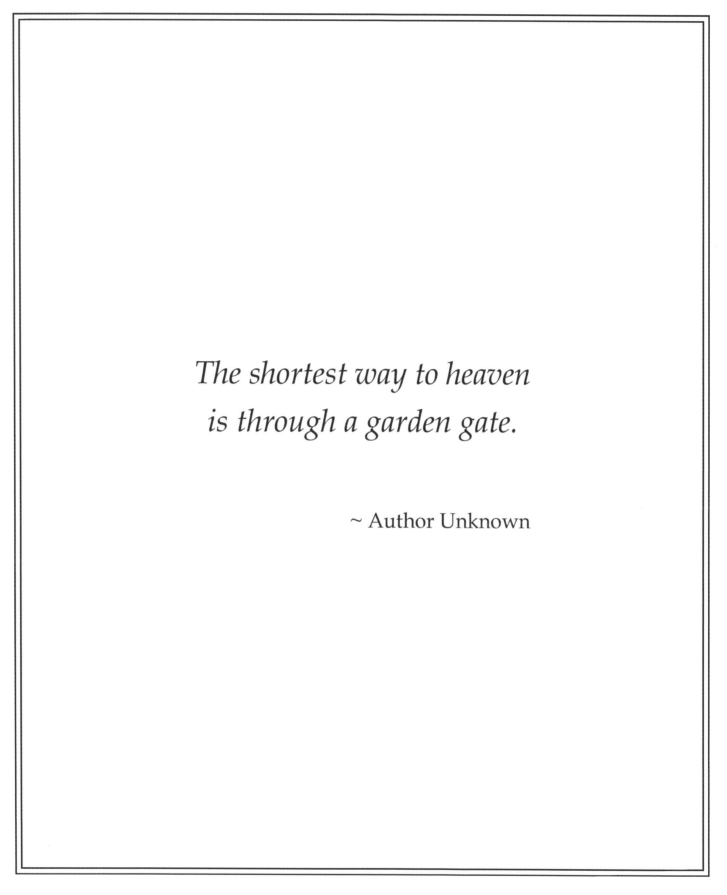

The shortest way to heaven
is through a garden gate.

~ Author Unknown

A gladiolus is also known as a "sword lily."

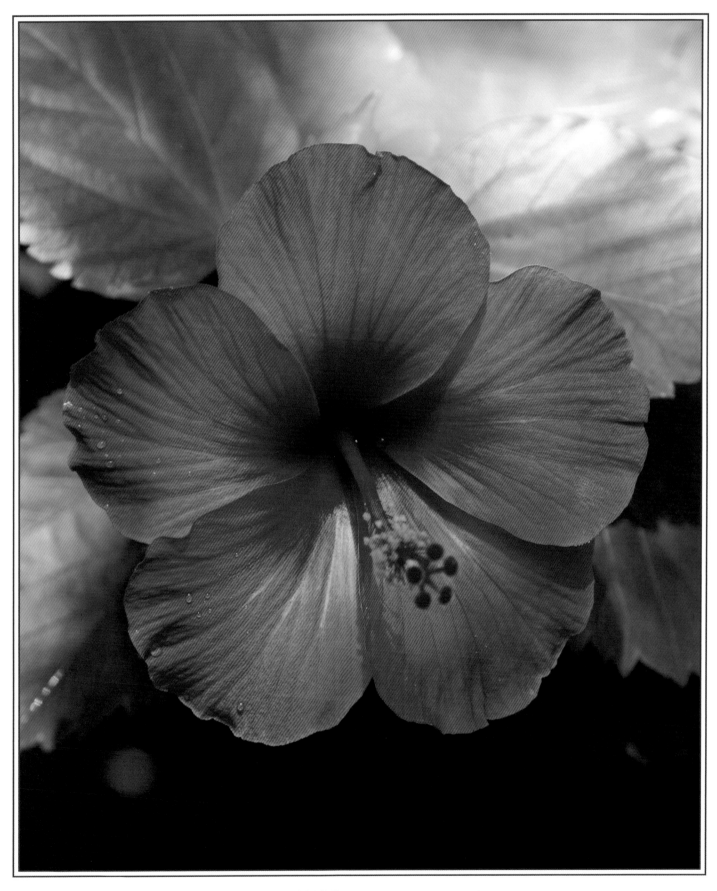

Hibiscus

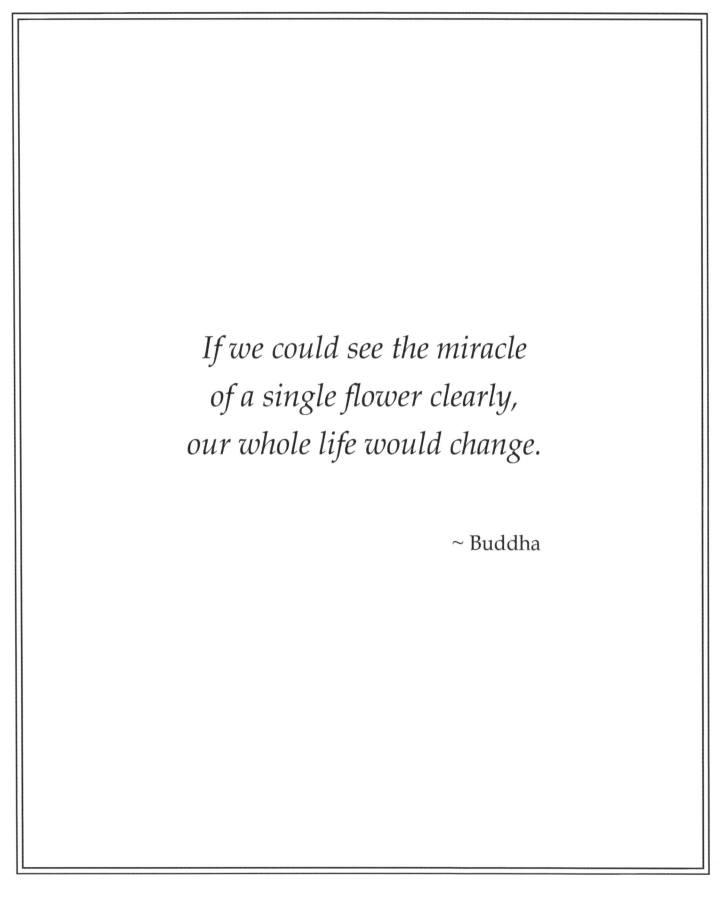

If we could see the miracle
of a single flower clearly,
our whole life would change.

~ Buddha

The hibiscus grows wild in many tropical regions around the world.

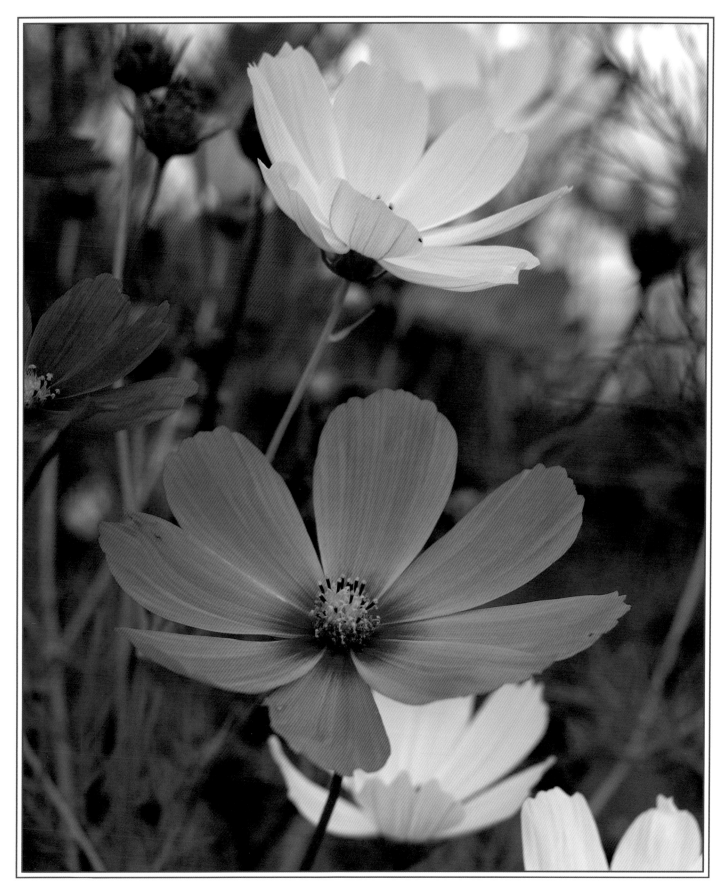

Cosmos

Happiness is to hold flowers in both hands.

~ Japanese Proverb

Cosmos attract butterflies and birds to a garden.

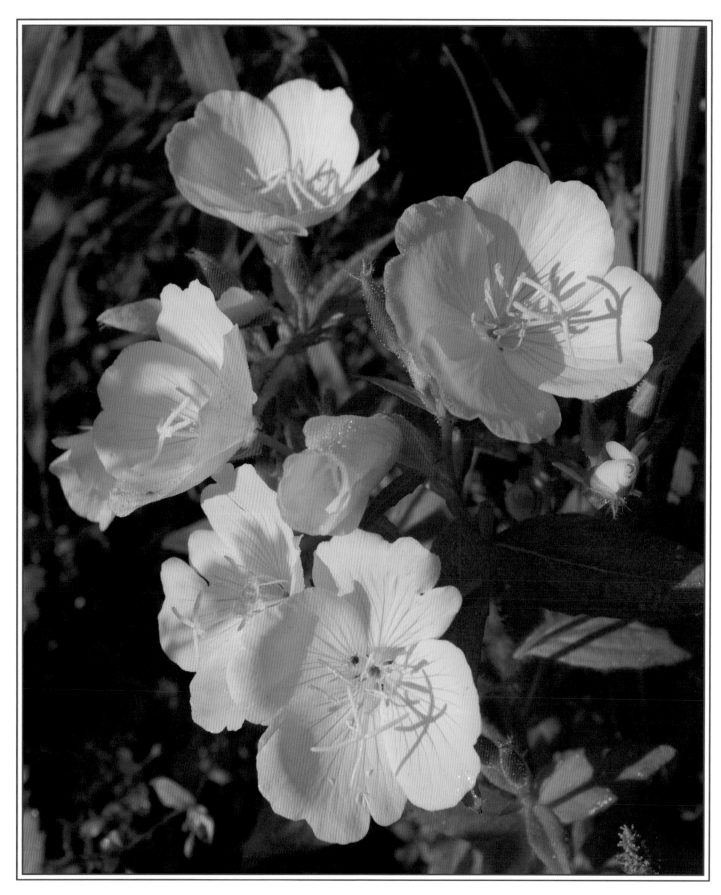

Evening Primrose

Everything has beauty,
but not everyone sees it.

~ Confucius

An evening primrose is also known as a "sun drop."

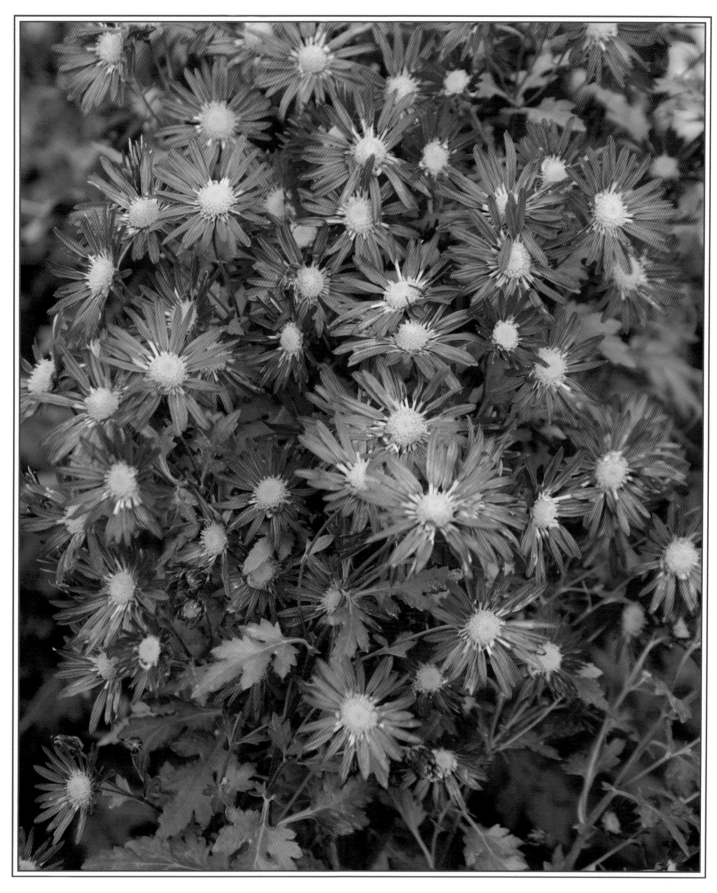

Chrysanthemum

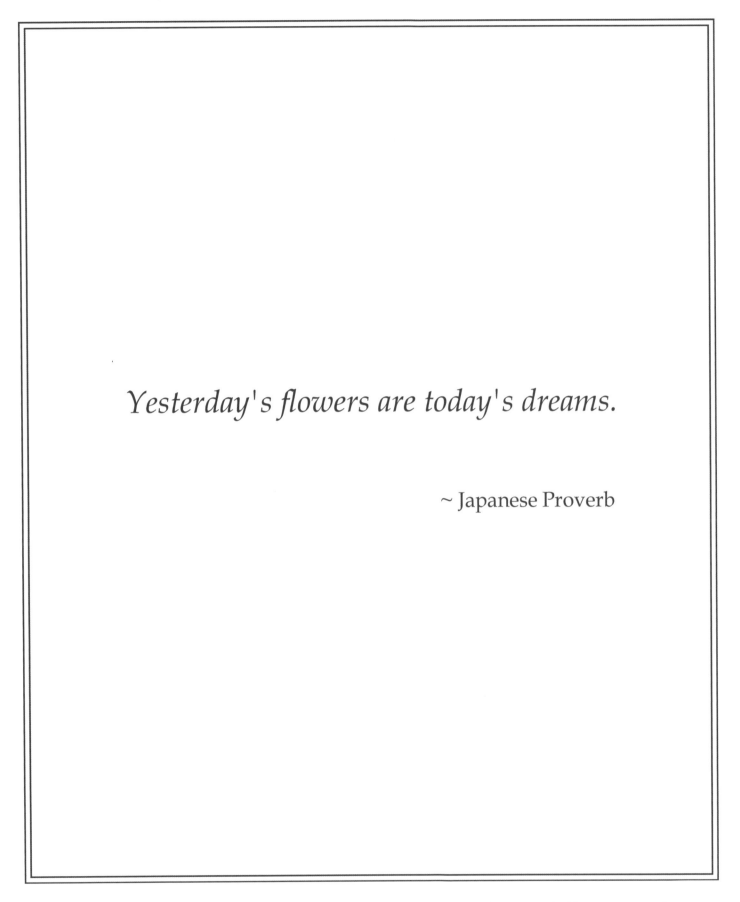

Yesterday's flowers are today's dreams.

~ Japanese Proverb

Chrysanthemums were brought to Japan by Buddhist monks.

Conversation Starters
and Activities

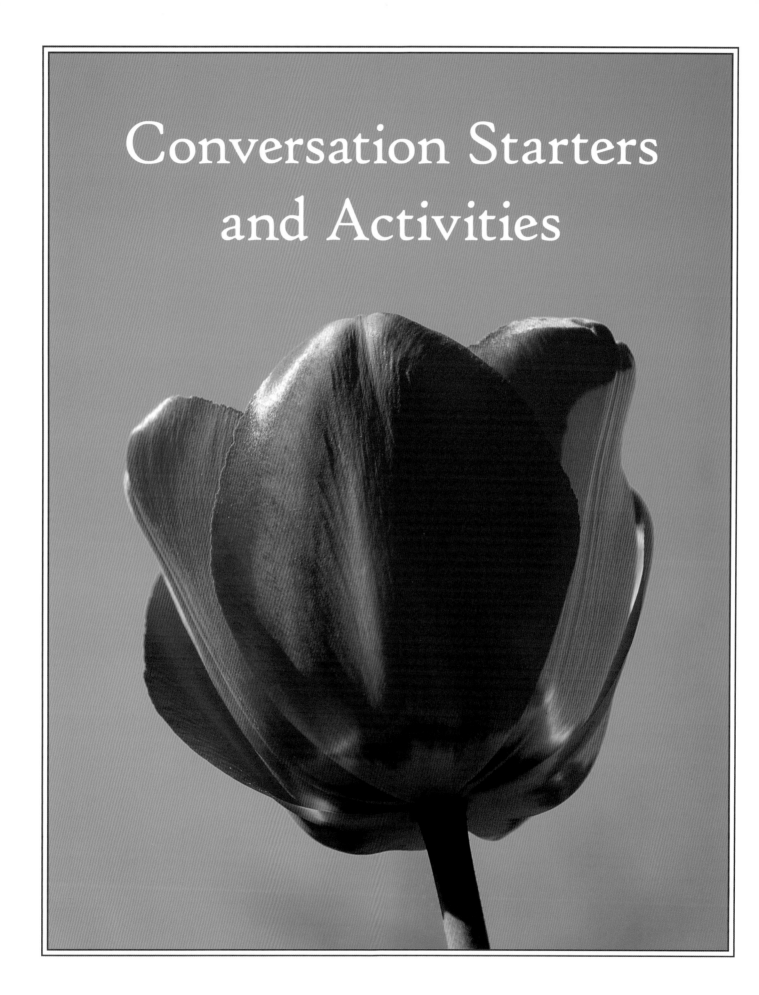

CONVERSATION STARTERS are designed to engage the user and encourage self-expression. They consist of a combination of close-ended (yes or no) and open-ended questions. Each series of four questions correlate to an individual set of pages and are intended to be referenced during the reading experience. Each question is designed to prompt a response by the user from a photograph, word, phrase, or idea from the STORY. After a response from a specific question, either verbal or nonverbal, encourage further discussion on that particular subject. Urging the user to elaborate on an experience allows them to connect to the story and to the caregiver.

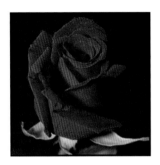

Did you know that the rose is the national flower of the United States?

Do you like roses?

Did your mother grow roses?

What is your favorite color rose?

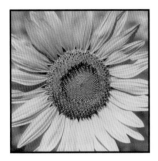

Did you know that the largest sunflower grew to be over 25-feet tall?

Did you ever stand next to a sunflower when you were a child?

Have you ever eaten sunflower seeds?

When you were a child, what did you want to be when you grew up?

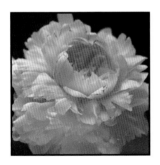

Did you know that peonies can live over one hundred years?

Have you ever grown peonies?

Do you like pink or white peonies?

What flowers do you like in a bouquet?

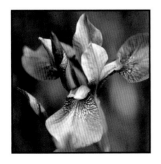

Did you know that the iris is the birthday flower for February?

Have you ever felt the velvety petals of an iris?

Have you ever been a member of a garden club?

What color irises have you seen in a garden?

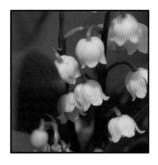

Did you know that the lily of the valley is the national flower of Yugoslavia?

Do you like the fragrance of lily of the valley?

Do you like to sit outdoors in the shade?

Where have you shopped for perfume?

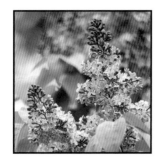

Did you know that most orchids are grown in tropical climates?

Do you like to sit outdoors on a sunny porch or patio?

Did your mother grow any flowers indoors?

For what occasions have you worn a corsage or boutonniere?

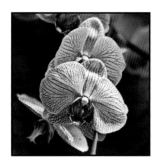

Did you know that the world's largest collection of lilacs is located in Rochester, New York?

Have you ever had a lilac bush?

Do you like the fragrance of lilacs?

Where did your mother put a vase of flowers in your childhood home?

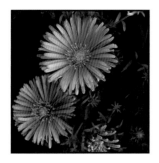

Did you know that the aster is the birthday flower for September?

Do you know anyone born in September?

Do asters remind you of autumn?

How did you prepare for the first day of school?

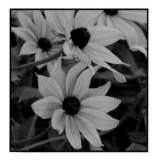

Did you know that the black-eyed Susan is the state flower of Maryland?

Do you know anyone named Susan?

Did you ever play in a field when you were a child?

What color are your eyes?

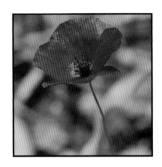

Did you know that in some countries artificial poppies are worn to remember those who served their country?

Have you ever bought a poppy from a veteran?

Have you ever baked anything with poppy seeds?

Who in your family served in the military?

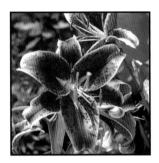

Did you know that lilies have blossoms shaped like trumpets?

Have you ever bought lilies from a florist?

Have you ever played a musical instrument?

What type of music do you enjoy?

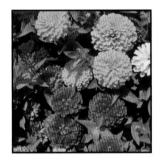

Did you know that a bouquet of zinnias means "thinking of friends"?

Do you like colorful flowers?

Have you ever seen a butterfly on a flower?

What did you and your friends like to do in the summer?

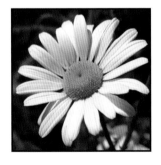

Did you know that Daisy was a very popular name for a girl in Victorian times?

Have you ever made a daisy chain?

Have you ever recited, "He loves me, he loves me not," as you picked the petals from a daisy?

What kind of flowers have you given to someone special?

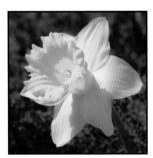

Did you know that over three million daffodils bloom on Nantucket Island, Massachusetts each spring?

Do you look forward to springtime?

Do daffodils bloom where you live?

What gardening chores did you do in the spring?

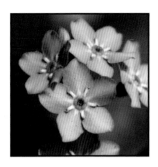

Did you know that the forget-me-not is the state flower of Alaska?

Have you ever been to Alaska?

Do you like the color blue?

What did you and your friends like to do in the winter?

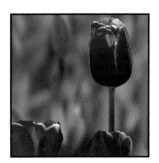

Did you know that the largest tulip festival in the United States is held in Holland, Michigan?

Have you ever planted spring bulbs?

Do you like red, yellow, or pink tulips?

What country did your ancestors emigrate from?

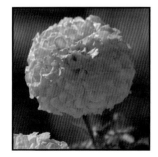

Did you know that the pansy is the traditional flower for a first wedding anniversary?

Have you ever picked a bouquet of pansies?

Do you like weddings?

Where did you go on your honeymoon?

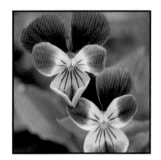

Did you know that there are over 100 varieties of hydrangeas?

Did your grandmother have a flower garden?

Have you ever dried or pressed flowers?

Where did your grandparents live?

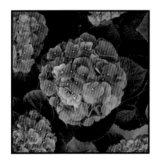

Did you know that marigolds are one of the most popular summer flowers?

Have you ever collected and saved seeds from flowers?

Have you ever watered flowers using a sprinkling can?

What kind of gardening tools have you used?

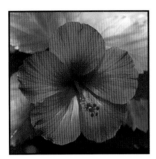

Did you know that the gladiolus is the birthday flower for August?

Do you enjoy the summer months?

Have you ever pulled weeds from a flower garden?

What was the weather like in August where you grew up?

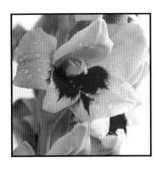

Did you know that the hibiscus is the state flower of Hawaii?

Have you ever taken a vacation to relax in the sun?

Have you ever worn a flower in your hair?

What tropical fruits do you like to eat?

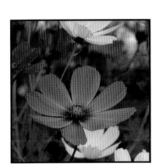

Did you know that cosmos grow in hot, sunny areas in Mexico?

Do you know how to speak Spanish?

Have you ever taken a trip to Mexico or South America?

What kind of Mexican foods do you like to eat?

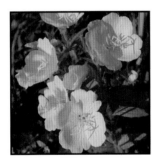

Did you know that the petals of the evening primrose open in the evening and close during the day?

Do you like to sit outside in the evening?

Do you enjoy watching a sunrise or sunset?

What did your family do together on summer evenings?

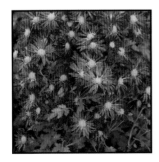

Did you know that the chrysanthemum is the birthday flower for November?

Have you ever bought mums at a greenhouse or garden center?

Do you enjoy the leaves changing color in the fall?

How did your family celebrate Thanksgiving when you were growing up?

ACTIVITIES are designed to enrich the user's life by introducing diversity into the daily routine through mental and physical engagement. They are intended to be performed under the supervision of a caregiver. Caution should be exercised when outdoors, in unfamiliar surroundings, or when using potentially harmful materials and/or equipment. Selection of an appropriate activity is dependent on individual ability; however, the user may participate or benefit from observing another individual perform the activity.

SENSORY STIMULATION ACTIVITIES

Create an indoor flower garden. Identify a location that receives bright sunlight in order to encourage healthy plants and abundant blooms. African violets, begonias, orchids, or amaryllises grow well indoors. Water the flowers regularly. Experience the vibrant colors and wonderful fragrances an indoor flower garden provides.

Dye a carnation. Fill a clear vase with water and add 10–20 drops of food coloring. Trim a white carnation's stem at an angle and place it in the vase. Check the carnation every few hours and monitor the colored water as it travels up the stem and transforms the petals of the flower.

Listen to "summer" music outdoors. Select popular music in a variety of genres, including classical, Hawaiian luau, beach music, and feel-good classics. Sing, whistle, hum, clap, or tap feet to the music. Enjoy the music outdoors in the warm summer air.

Inspect flowers with a magnifying glass. Gather a variety of flowers and study the petals, leaves, stems, seeds, etc. Compare the size, color, shape, and texture of each flower. Discover the wonder of nature close up.

Collect seeds from flowers. After blooming, remove the seed heads from the plants. Place them in a paper bag, close the bag loosely, hang it upside down, and allow the seeds to dry for several days. Next, transfer the seeds to a paper plate and allow them to dry for several more days. Place the seeds in an airtight container, label them, and store them in a cool, dry place.

Make a dried-flower arrangement. Bunch fresh flowers into a bouquet and tie a string around the stems. Hang the bouquet, blossoms down, in a dark, warm, dry place. Allow it to dry for four weeks. Arrange the dried flowers in a vase and enjoy their beauty.

Moisturize hands with floral-scented lotion. Play relaxing music and turn on a flameless luminary to create a calming atmosphere. Gently massage hands and arms with a lavender or rose-scented lotion. Savor the serene setting as the lotion soothes the skin.

Build a terrarium. Choose a clear plastic or glass container and fill the bottom with pebbles for drainage. Add topsoil, plant mosses and plants in the container, and water as needed. Add decorative items such as small figurines, plastic bugs, jewelry, stones, beads, etc. Enjoy the terrarium garden indoors year round.

CREATIVE EXPRESSION ACTIVITIES

Make pressed flowers. Flowers that are flat such as violets, cosmos, and pansies work best for pressing. Place the flowers between sheets of newspaper. Put the newspaper and flowers between the pages of a thick book. Leave undisturbed for 2–3 weeks. When the flowers are flat and dry, they can be used in a variety of creative projects.

Paint a still life. Put a single flower in a vase and place it on a table where it can be easily viewed. Paint the background and allow it to dry. Sketch a light outline of the flower and vase in pencil. Begin painting the largest parts of the still life and then focus on the detail. Work with light tones first, then with dark tones. Allow the painting to dry completely before displaying it.

Photograph flowers. Use a disposable or digital camera. Choose a subject. Consider a single flower, a group of flowers, or a field of flowers. Walk around the subject and look for the best angle and lighting. Print the photos and share them with family and friends.

Paint a clay pot. Draw a design or pattern on a pot with a pencil. Fill in the design with markers or paints. Cover the outside of the pot with shellac to protect the artwork. Plant marigolds or petunias in the pot and enjoy the beauty of the flowers and the pot.

Create a flower scrapbook. Collect photographs, pictures, pressed flowers, seed packets, etc. Arrange the items on the pages and adhere them using a glue stick. Write a brief description on each page. Add embellishments such as stickers, rub-ons, metal accents, etc. Put the finished pages in page protectors, place them in an album, and share it with family and friends.

PHYSICAL MOVEMENT ACTIVITIES

Plant flower bulbs. When choosing bulbs, consider the colors and size of the blooms for the space. Spring flower bulbs can be planted in the late summer and fall. Plant the hyacinths, tulips, daffodils, etc. with the pointed end of the bulb up. Fertilize, water as needed, and enjoy the splash of color the flowers bring to a garden in the spring.

Clean and oil gardening tools. Remove soil or other residue from the tools. A wire brush is good for removing rust and stubborn soil. Wipe the metal areas with oil and lubricate the moving parts. Caring for garden tools will protect them during winter storage.

Visit a botanical garden. A public garden is a beautiful place and a visit can inspire an even greater appreciation for plants and flowers. Walk through a variety of indoor and outdoor displays. Experience the rich, varied colors and the wonderful scents of the plant collections.

Plant a butterfly garden. Butterflies are attracted to flowers with bright colors and strong scents. Plant purple coneflowers, lantanas, asters, goldenrod, or milkweed. Purchase a book about butterflies and identify the species that are attracted to the garden.